PALEO DIET COOKBOOK

Discover the Benefits of the Paleo Diet and Start Losing
Weight Today

(A Paleo Cookbook You Won't Be Able to Put Down)

Florence Abrams

Published by Alex Howard

Florence Abrams

Paleo Diet Cookbook: Discover the Benefits of the Paleo Diet and Start Losing Weight Today (A Paleo Cookbook You Won't Be Able to Put Down)

ISBN 978-1-77485-025-1

Legal & Disclaimer

The information contained in this book is not designed to replace or take the place of any form of medicine or professional medical advice. The information in this book has been provided for educational and entertainment purposes only.

The information contained in this book has been compiled from sources deemed reliable, and it is accurate to the best of the Author's knowledge; however, the Author cannot guarantee its accuracy and validity and cannot be held liable for any errors or omissions. Changes are periodically made to this book. You must consult your doctor or get professional medical advice before using any of the suggested remedies, techniques, or information in this book.

Upon using the information contained in this book, you agree to hold harmless the Author from and against any damages, costs, and expenses, including any legal fees potentially resulting from the application of any of the information provided by this guide. This disclaimer applies to any damages or injury caused by the use and application, whether directly or indirectly, of any advice or information presented, whether for breach of contract, tort, negligence, personal injury, criminal intent, or under any other cause of action.

You agree to accept all risks of using the information presented inside this book. You need to consult a professional medical practitioner in order to ensure you are both able and healthy enough to participate in this program.

Table of Contents

Part 1

Introduction

Weight loss on the Paleo diet is not only possible, it is inevitable! Present day eating habits are not healthy and our bodies are not designed to generate energy from the majority of foods that we eat. Most of the foods that we consume are not natural though we might label some of them as being healthy and nutritious.

After a few years of eating the way I was told to by the food gurus the majority of us do I started to put on weight. Keeping that weight on for many years, All along the way, carrying that extra poundage around and genuinely not feeling incredible, I decided to retreat to the way I was taught to eat. Which of course (and I didn't know it) was the Paleo Diet. Within a few short weeks (5or6) I lost 50 pounds.

There are several health benefits offered by the Paleo diet. Studies reveal that this diet is extremely helpful in losing weight, but it also acts as prevention for medical conditions such as cardiovascular disease, cancer, hypertension, and osteoporosis.

This unique diet plan focuses on losing weight, building muscle, and staying fit and healthy. The diet of the caveman included only fresh and naturally occurring foods which lead them to be strong and able to endure a lot of hardships.

The Paleo diet is sometimes identified as the caveman diet or the diet eaten by Palaeolithic man, i.e. people living anywhere from 10,000 to 2,500,000 years ago. The fundamental idea of the paleo diet is to replicate the diet of our forebears, who were classed as hunters and gatherers. Trying out a paleo lifestyle will probably be difficult sometimes, as many of the favorite food consumed by the western populous are not listed on the paleo diet regime. The modern Paleo Diet.

Before we get too depressed at the thought of having no idea what the paleo diet actually was, what do we actually mean when we say we're going paleo or following a paleo recipe?

Again there's a simple and a slightly lengthier explanation. In brief, then, on a paleo diet we eat nothing that Paleolithic peoples wouldn't have eaten and as much as possible of what they would have consumed.

What does that mean in real, food on plate, terms? Plenty of vegetables, eggs, some meat and fish and some fruit, nuts and seeds really. That's about it. To put it another way, no grains, no refined sugars or sweeteners, no legumes, no potatoes, no dairy, no preservatives, additives, processed, emulsified, manufactured junk!

Another way of looking at it is that if you can't eat it raw then you probably shouldn't be eating it at all. You might not want to eat a raw food diet but you'll find that most everything on a paleo diet could be eaten raw if necessary. Veggies, fruits, nuts and seeds and yes, meat and fish can all be eaten raw. As mentioned, you might not want to chew on raw meat or fish, but you'll do a lot better with that than with raw potatoes or wheat for example.

Though sticking to such a diet might be difficult for some, it definitely fits our human genetics much better than our modern, chemical-filled diet. As far as weight loss goes, the Paleo diet was followed naturally by our ancestors and has been proven to be one of the best diets for a healthy lifestyle.

Benefits of the Paleo Diet

The advantages of the Paleo Diet have been researched and proven in numerous academic journals. It is amazing how changing what we put in our mouths can cause dramatic changes in our quality of life.

Lose fat- Though the Paleo diet is designed as a weight loss plan people inherently lose weight. The foods that make up the Paleo diet are what we call fat burning foods. In fact, the Paleo diet allows you to eat large quantities of delicious food while restricting calories. The result is a lean, fit body.

- **Improve Digestion**- Many digestive problems such as, irritable bowel syndrome, Crohn's disease and indigestion can be avoided.

- **Combats Acne**– Eating the Paleo way means avoiding the foods that cause acne. When sebum is overproduced or obstructed the sebaceous glands enlarge and form pimples. Foods in the Paleo diet do not cause the insulin spikes that cause a sebum boost. As a result, you can expect smoother, more attractive skin.

- **Feel Great!** - Not only does the Paleo diet help people healthier and look younger it also makes you feel better. Paleo supporters swear by the caveman lifestyle because it just "feels" right. The only way to find out the energy and confidence they experience is to try it for yourself.

- **Fight Disease**- The Paleo diet is proven to help prevent diabetes, Parkinson's avoid Parkinson's, cancer, heart disease and strokes.

Diet Basics

People assume the Paleo Diet is complicated are difficult to follow. It is actually quite simple. Eat real foods. For a guideline on portions, 56–65% of your calories should come from animals, 36–45% from plant based foods. Keep proteins high at 19-35% carbohydrates at 22-40% and fat at 28-58%.

Tips for the Paleo Lifestyle

Unfortunately, the cheapest and quickest foods available today are usually the least nutritious. Our busy lifestyles have our kids raised on an eating processed and fast foods. The popular tradition even makes having real foods the odd concept. Actually knowing the tested benefits, some refuse to attempt the Paleo diet plan because they still find it too difficult. Living a good, healthy fulfilling life is worth a few modest changes. Maintaining a Paleo life style is realistic with a few tips.

- **Stay Organized**- The number one tip is to be organized and prepared. The biggest challenge will be to have Paleo foods available at your home and plan your meals. You are much more likely to eat healthy food choices if it is readily available at home.
- **Change How You Shop**- Find the best farmers markets, butchers and grocery stores in your area. Before going to the grocery have a list of items you plan to pick up. Also, shop the perimeter of grocery stores to avoid the aisles filled with processed foods. This may be difficult at first, but after a month or so you will know longer feel a need to peruse the sugar aisles.
- **Clean Your Pantry**- Clear your cupboards of all the cereals, pasta, and processed foods in your cabinets. Don't worry. You will replace these foods with much more satisfying fresh and healthy foods.
- **Learn to Work the Kitchen**- Unlike a diet based on grains, there are many foods to eat on the Paleo Diet you should never become bored. The best way to take advantage of everything nature has to offer is to learn how to cook. By combining the diverse flavors, there is an endless amount of tasty dishes to excite your taste buds.
- **Dress Your Food**- Most of the condiments on the store shelves are filled with preservatives. However, you can enhance the flavor of your foods by making your own condiments at home. Ketchup, mustard, salad dressings and sauces can be made at home naturally with delicious results.
- **Exercise**- Just changing your eating habits will cause you to lose weight naturally on the Paleo Diet. Add exercise to the mix, and you will be amazed at how quickly you notice a difference. Your true, toned physique will come out as pounds shed. You will also notice the amount of energy increased compared to when you ate a traditional diet. Start feeling strong, energetic, mentally sharper and all around younger.

- **Join Support System**- Find chat rooms and forums where like-minded people meet. Participate at a gym where the Paleo Diet is the main lifestyle choice. It is nice to share ideas on the best Paleo books, and even give advice on keeping true to the diet plan. Joining a community online or in person is extremely motivating when you learn about how the other member's lives improved just from staying true to the Paleo way.

1. Breakfast Muffins

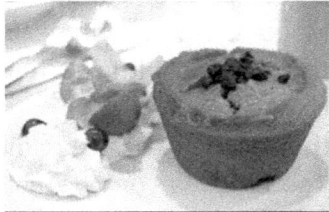

1.1. Banana Carrot Muffins

Yields: 12-14 muffins

Ingredients

Dry Ingredients:
1 1/4 cup almond flour
1/2 tsp baking soda
1/2 tsp baking powder
1/2 tsp salt
1 tbsp. cinnamon
1/2 tsp allspice
Wet Ingredients:
3 eggs - whisked

2 bananas - mashed
1/2 cup almond butter
1/3 cup raw honey
1/4 cup coconut oil
1 tsp vanilla extract

Fold In:
1 cup grated carrot
1/2 cup chopped walnuts, pecans or raisins

Instructions

1. Pre-heat stove to 350º F.
2. In a large blending bowl, blend all the dry ingredients.
3. In another mid-size bowl, merge all wet ingredients.
4. Add the wet ingredients into the dry ingredients bowl and blend nicely.
5. Then fold grated carrots and the walnuts, pecans or raisins into the batter.
6. Put batter into lined muffin tin molds (utilize paper or silicone cup liners) Fill up each cup around two-thirds full.
7. Bake 22-25 minutes, or until an injected toothpick comes out thoroughly clean
Cool and enjoy!

1.2. Just Peachy Morning Muffins

Yield: 8-9 muffins

Ingredients

1 cup peeled and diced fresh peaches
200 grams almond flour (about 2 cups)
½ teaspoon baking soda
⅛ Teaspoon sea salt, fine ground
3 eggs
2 tablespoons ghee, melted
2 tablespoons honey
1 tablespoon lemon juice

Instructions

1. Preheat stove to 325 degrees Fahrenheit and grease or line muffin tin.
2. Mix dry ingredients in big bowl. Blend wet ingredients in mid-size bowl. Mix wet ingredients into dry ingredients and delicately fold in peaches.
3. Utilize a sizable ice cream or cookie scoop to fill up muffin cups ¾ full.
4. Bake for 25 - 30 minutes, or until golden brown and toothpick entered in center comes out thoroughly clean. Cool on wire rack.

1.3. Pumpkin Muffins

Yield: 12 muffins

Ingredients
1/2 c Coconut Flour
1/2 t Salt
1/2 t Baking Soda
1/2 t Baking Powder
5 Eggs
2 Egg Whites
1 Large Mashed Banana
1/2 c Almond Butter (or Coconut Manna for nut-free)
1 t Vanilla
1 1/2 t Cinnamon
3 T Honey
1 Apple, any color, roughly chopped

Instructions
1. Mix all of the ingredients except for the apple in a sizable blending bowl and merge to combine.
2. Whisk on high speed with an electrical mixing machine for 3 minutes, until good and fluffy. Fold in the apples. Spoon into prepared muffin tins.
3. Bake at 350 degrees Fahrenheit for 20 minutes. Some may continue to be slightly gooey due to the apple, but that's exactly what we want!
4. Cool down completely before removing from muffin pan.

1.4. Scrumptious Blueberry Muffins

Yields: 10 muffins

Ingredients

2 1/2 cups almond flour
1 Tablespoon coconut flour
1/4 teaspoon salt
1/2 teaspoon baking soda
1 Tablespoon vanilla
1/4 cup coconut oil
1/4 cup maple syrup
1/4 cup coconut milk*
2 eggs
1 cup fresh or frozen blueberries
2-3 Tablespoons cinnamon

Instructions

1. Pre-heat stove to 350 degrees.
2. Line a 12 count muffin tin and slightly oil with coconut oil.
3. In a blending bowl blend together almond flour, coconut flour, salt, and baking soda and mix to combine.
4. Add in coconut oil, eggs, maple syrup, coconut milk, and vanilla; mix nicely.
5. Fold in blueberries and include cinnamon.
6. Disperse into muffin tin.
7. Sprinkle with extra cinnamon.
8. Bake for 22-25 minutes. Allow to cool down and enjoy!

1.5. Walnut And Banana Muffins

Yield: 6-10 muffins

Ingredients

3 large eggs
¼ cup coconut oil
2 medium bananas
3 dates, pitted
10 drops stevia
¼ cup coconut flour
¼ teaspoon Celtic sea salt
½ teaspoon baking soda
½ cup walnuts, toasted and chopped

Instructions

1. Set eggs, oil, bananas, dates and stevia in a blender; mix on medium speed until merged.
2. Put in coconut flour, salt and baking soda and mix until smooth.
3. Fold in walnuts.
4. Scoop ¼ cup batter into a lined muffin pan.
5. Bake at 350° for 20-25 minutes.
6. Cool off and serve up.

Nutrition Facts
Serving Size 53 g

Amount Per Serving
Calories 135   Calories from Fat 94

% Daily Value*

Total Fat 10.7g — 16%
Saturated Fat 3.4g — 27%
Cholesterol 54mg — 18%
Sodium 84mg — 4%
Potassium 154mg — 4%
Total Carbohydrates 6.5g — 3%
Dietary Fiber 1.2g — 5%
Sugars 4.1g

Protein 3.1g

Vitamin A 2% • Vitamin C 4%
Calcium 1% • Iron 3%

Nutrition Grade B-
* Based on a 2000 calorie diet

Nutritional Analysis

Bad points
• High in saturated fat
• High in cholesterol

2. Breakfast Omelets

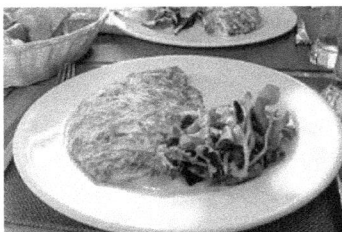

2.1. Sweet Potato and Bacon Omelet

Yield: 3 Servings

Ingredients

Sweet Potato-Ingredients

1 1/2 cup diced sweet potato (1-2cm chunks)
1 small white onion, cut in half and sliced roughly
A few springs of fresh thyme
A pinch of sea salt
1 tbsp. coconut oil

Other Ingredients

3-4 rashers of bacon, including the short cut part
6 eggs, whisked
A pinch of black pepper
A little ghee or coconut oil
A little crumbled goats cheese
Mixed salad greens & sliced cucumber

Instructions

1. Preheat stove to 350 degrees.

2. Brush the bottom of a cooking tray with coconut oil or allow it melt instantly in the oven.

3. Place sweet potato, onion and fresh thyme leaves in a tray and roast in the oven for 20-30 minutes. Stir a few times after the first 15 minutes of roasting.

4. Spread with a bit of salt towards the end.

5. Trim away the rind of the bacon but don't throw away.

6. Chop bacon, as well as the fat in the streaky rushes, into little cubes. Cut the rind pieces into 3-4 pieces.

7. Heat up a bit of ghee or coconut oil in a frying pan you are going to be cooking the omelet in. Fry bacon for 5 minutes, stirring repeatedly, until it's brown and crispy. After that turn the heat to medium.

8. Put in sweet potato blend and stir through until heated up. Pour whisked egg mix over potato and bacon ensuring the whole surface area is evenly covered.

9. Cook for approximately 4-5 minutes or until the egg is set and cooked throughout, you can cover up the pan with a lid to speed up the cooking process.

10. Half way through, distribute some broken goats cheese and black pepper. Once again, cheese is optional.

Serve up with a side salad of mixed greens, cucumber, lemon juice & olive oil.

2.2. Avocado Bacon Omelet

Yield: 2 servings

Ingredients

4 bacon slices

1 avocado
2 tbsp. minced red onion
1 tbsp. minced fresh cilantro
1 dash hot sauce
4 eggs

Instructions

1. Cook bacon until crispy.
2. At the same time as bacon is cooking, cut your avocado in half, take away the pit, and scoop the flesh into a bowl. Smash it up, but not too fine—a bit of texture is good.
3. Insert onion and cilantro to avocado. Whenever the bacon is completed, drain it and crumble or cut it in, too. Blend it all up.
4. At this point make your omelets, one by one. Make use of half the avocado mixture in each one. Top with additional hot sauce, if preferred.

2.3. Omelet Ham Muffins

Yield: 8 servings

Ingredients

8 eggs
8 ounces cooked ham, crumbled
1 cup diced red bell pepper
1 cup diced onion
1/4 teaspoon salt
1/8 teaspoon ground black pepper
2 tablespoons water

Instructions

1. Preheat stove to 350 degrees Fahrenheit F (175 degrees C). Oil 8 muffin cups or line with paper liners.

2. Beat eggs collectively in a sizable bowl. Combine ham, bell pepper, onion, salt, black pepper, and water into the beaten eggs. Fill egg combination evenly into prepared muffin cups.

3. Bake in the preheated stove until muffins are set in the middle, 18 to 20 minutes.

2.4. Spinach Omelet

Yield: 1 serving

Ingredients

2 eggs
1.5 cups raw spinach
Coconut oil, about 1 tbsp.
1/3 c salsa
1 tbsp. fresh cilantro

Instructions

1. Melt coconut oil on medium temperature in frying pan.
2. Put in spinach, cook until generally wilted. Whip eggs and include in pan. (Other recommended ingredients- peppers, mushrooms, cheese, etc. . .)

3. Turn once the egg sets around the edges. As soon as it's virtually done include the salsa on top simply to warm it.
4. Transfer to plate and top with cilantro.

2.5. Easy Onion Omelet

Yield: 1-2 servings

Ingredients

1 tablespoon your choice of fat
1 cup onions, chopped
Coarse ground sea salt, to taste
Coarse ground black pepper, to taste
4 large organic eggs

Instructions

1. Include your selection of cooking oil, I used grass-fed butter, to a medium-size skillet over moderate heat.
2. Once butter is melted, insert onions to the skillet. Sauté onions until tender.
3. While onions are cooking, break eggs into a compact bowl and whisk.
4. Whenever onions are translucent and aromatic, include eggs to the pan.
5. Place a lid on and let it cook for 1-2 minutes.
6. Check up on omelet and turn one half over the other.
7. Cover up pan with the lid and cook until eggs are completed. Make sure to remain close and monitor it.

8. Decrease heat when necessary to medium-low.

9. As soon as eggs are solid, switch off heat, move the omelet to a plate and serve up.

3. Breakfast Casseroles

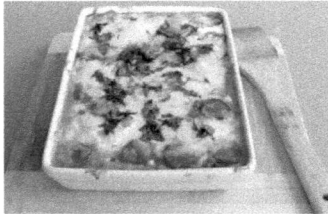

3.1. Breakfast Low-Carb Casserole

Yield 6-10 servings

Ingredients

Softened ghee, for greasing the slow cooker
1/2 pound bulk breakfast sausage, crumbled
6 ounces bacon, chopped
1/2 cup yellow onion, diced
1 pound white sweet potatoes, peeled and shredded
1 red bell pepper, seeded and diced
1 orange bell pepper, seeded and diced
16 large eggs, beaten
1/2 cup almond milk
1/4 cup full-fat coconut milk
1 teaspoon sea salt
3/4 teaspoon dry mustard
1/4 teaspoon cracked black pepper
Green onions, for garnish

Instructions

1. Oil a slow-cooker insert nicely with palm shortening or softened ghee.

2. Cook the sausage, bacon, and onion in a skillet over medium-high temperature for 10 to 12 minutes, until the sausage is browned also the onion is softened.

3. Drain off the unwanted fats.

4. Position the shredded sweet potatoes in the slow cooker, and push them down slightly.

5. Put in the meat and onion mix and the bell peppers to the slow cooker.

6. In a big bowl, whisk collectively the eggs, milks, salt, mustard, and pepper. Add into the slow cooker.

7. Cover up and cook on low for 6 to 8 hours.

3.2. Simple Casserole Chorizo

Yield: 3-4 servings

Ingredients

1lb chorizo (or other ground meat)
10 organic eggs
1/2 green bell pepper, chopped
1-2 cups onion, chopped
Coarse ground sea salt, to taste
Coarse ground black pepper, to taste
Dried oregano, to taste
Fresh dill, minced

Instructions

1. Pre-heat the stove to 350° Fahrenheit.

2. Brown the chorizo in a skillet over moderate heat, for roughly 8-10 minutes.

3. Whisk eggs in a large blending bowl.

4. Insert the green pepper, onion, sea salt, black pepper and oregano to eggs. Whisk to intermix.

5. Combine the chorizo to mix and stir again to intermix.

6. Fill the egg combination into a 2 .2 quart oblong glass baking dish. Dab the whole thing with a layer of fresh minced dill.

7. Bake for 30 minutes or until the middle has set. (Check utilizing a toothpick.)

3.3. Breakfast Sausage And Sweet Potato Casserole

Serves 8-10 servings

Ingredients

1 1/2 lbs. breakfast sausage
1/2 tbsp. coconut oil
12 eggs
2 sweet potatoes, peeled and diced
1/2 large sweet onion, diced
1 tsp garlic powder
1/4 tsp nutmeg
1 tip sea salt
1 tsp pepper
1/4 cup coconut milk
4 cups power greens (kale, spinach, arugula)

Instructions

1. Heat up stove to 375 degrees Fahrenheit.

2. In a sizable skillet over moderate heat, melt coconut oil and put in sausage.

3. Brown and break separately with a wooden spoon.

4. Whisk eggs in additionally sizable bowl. .

5. Cut up sweet potatoes and onion in your food processor. Combine into eggs with seasoning, coconut milk and power greens.

6. Oil 9x13 casserole dish with additional coconut oil.

7. Add in egg mixture and blend in sausage.

8. Cook for 45 minutes. Cover up with foil and cook for 10 more minutes or until middle is set.

3.4. Delightful Bacon W/ Kale Casserole

Yield: 4 servings

Ingredients

1 tablespoon Olive Oil
3 cups chop Kale
½ cups cook and dice Bacon
10 individual Egg
⅛ Teaspoons Salt
⅛ Teaspoons Black Pepper

Instructions

1. Heat up oil in a frying pan and sauté kale until soft (approximately 3-4 minutes).

2. Separate and layer kale and bacon in suggested selection of greased 8x8 aluminum foil pan.

3. Break eggs into a sizable bowl. Whisk all together and season with salt and pepper.

4. Add over ingredients in the pan.

5. Bake at 375 degrees Fahrenheit for 20 to 25 minutes until middle is set and top part is lightly browned.

3.5. On The Range Chicken Casserole

Yield: 2-4 servings

Ingredients

2 cups shredded cooked chicken
1 1/3 cups cooked and mashed butternut squash
1/4 cup coconut cream (the thick stuff from the top of a can of coconut milk. Don't shake the can) OR substitute yogurt or sour cream
1/4 cup ghee or butter or coconut oil (coconut oil will impart a stronger coconut taste)
1 cup thawed green peas
1 tsp. Herbamare seasoning salt or Real Salt Seasoning Salt or your favorite seasoning salt
1 - 2 Tbs. raw apple cider vinegar (Bragg's)
Optional: 1/2 cup unsweetened shredded coconut for the topping

Instructions

1. Add all the ingredients in a saucepan and cook over medium temperature until the peas are heated through and things are all melty and creamy.

2. Sprinkle with toasted coconut, if preferred.

3. If you would like, toast the coconut in a skillet over medium temperature. Stir until golden and toasty which usually takes a matter of minutes.

4. Breakfast Waffles

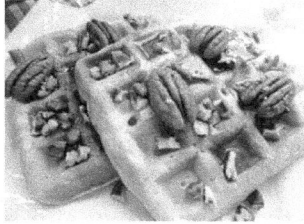

4.1. Cinnamon-Banana Waffles

Yield: 4-6 servings

Ingredients

WAFFLES
4 large eggs, room temperature
1 large ripe banana 1 cup full fat coconut milk
1/3 cup coconut oil, warmed if solid 2 tsp. vanilla extract
 2 Tbsp. raw honey
1/2 cup coconut flour
1/4 cup blanched almond flour
1/2 cup + 2 Tbsp. tapioca flour
2 tsp. ground cinnamon
1 tsp. sea salt
Melted coconut oil (to grease waffle iron)

HONEY CINNAMON SYRUP
1/2 cup coconut oil, warmed if solid
1/2 cup raw honey, warmed if solid
2 tsp. vanilla extract
2 tsp. ground cinnamon

Sliced bananas (optional topping)

Instructions

1. Blend all of the waffle ingredients in a blender and mix until smooth. Enable the batter to sit for approximately 10 minutes and then blend again for about 3 seconds before utilizing.
2. Coat your waffle iron with a bit of bit of coconut oil to avoid everything from sticking.
3. Fill enough batter to simply cover the bottom of the waffle maker, shut and cook until light brown. Each waffle maker will vary by size and cooking time so watch the waffles to make sure they do not burn up.

HONEY CINNAMON SYRUP:
1. Melt all of the topping ingredients together in a little saucepan and stir until just combined.
2. Drizzle over waffles, top with chopped up bananas (are optional) and enjoy!

4.2. Pecans And Banana Waffles

Yield: 3-4 waffles

Ingredients

1 1/2 cups almond flour
5 eggs (mine were on the small side, so 4 large ones may be fine)
1/4 teaspoon baking soda
1/4 teaspoon salt

2 ripe bananas, mashed (the more ripe they are, the sweeter the waffles will be)
1/2 teaspoon pumpkin pie spice
1/2 teaspoon cinnamon
1 teaspoon vanilla extract
Coconut oil
Chopped pecans

Instructions

1. Pre- heat your waffle iron.

2. At the same time, blend all of your ingredients together, besides the coconut oil and pecans.

3. As soon as the waffle iron is heated, drop a small amount of coconut oil in each square.

4. Scatter some or each of them with chopped pecans.

5. Pay close attention to the waffle iron to make sure your waffles aren't burning.

6. Remove the waffles out and enjoy!

You can add on some organic fruit spread or a homemade whipped cream topping.

4.3. Sweet Potato Waffles

Yield: 3-4 waffles

Ingredients

2 cups sweet potato puree (about 2 large sweet potatoes worth)
4 eggs
2 tablespoons coconut flour
1 teaspoon baking powder
1 teaspoon vanilla
1 teaspoon cinnamon
1/4 teaspoon Chinese 5-spice or allspice
A dash of cloves
A mister with coconut oil or butter for greasing the waffle maker

Instructions

1. In a sizable blending bowl, blend all of the ingredients while heating up the waffle iron.

2. Oil waffle iron or spray with coconut oil or butter, completely coating to prevent sticking.

3. Fill batter into the middle, leaving behind about 1 .5 inches clear around the side of the waffle iron. Close up iron and prepare until done.

4. Serve with maple syrup, apple sauce, almond butter or other preferred toppings.

4.4. Waffles With Caramelized Apple Syrup

Yield: 4-6 waffles

Ingredients

3 large eggs
¾ cup whole macadamia nuts or raw cashews
¼ cup raw pecans
¼ cup unsweetened almond milk or coconut milk
3 tablespoon coconut oil, melted
2 tablespoon honey
¼ cup coconut flour
¾ teaspoon baking soda
¼ teaspoon sea salt
2 teaspoon pumpkin pie spice

Caramelized Apple Syrup
3 tablespoon unsalted grass-fed butter, ghee, or palm shortening
¼ cup honey, preferably light in color
1 lb. baking apples – peeled, cored, and diced
¼ cup coconut milk
Pinch of sea salt

Instructions

Waffles

1. Pre-heat a waffle iron.

2. Mix the eggs, macadamia nuts, pecans, milk, honey, and melted coconut oil in a blender.

3. Mix until very smooth and creamy. If desired, stop the mixer and push the combination down the edges with a spatula to ensure an even blend.

4. Place the salt, baking soda, and coconut flour, and blend once more for approximately 30 seconds until completely incorporated.

5. If the waffle iron needs oil, dispersed a little coconut oil on each side.

6. Fill the batter into the waffle iron so that it just covers the lower portion of the iron , remaining cautious not to overfill as these do rise a lot and may spill over .

7. Make the waffles until the waffle iron has stopped steaming, about 45 seconds. Every waffle iron may be different in cook times.

8. Replicate until the batter has been utilized up.

9. Serve up hot with caramelized apple syrup.

Syrup
1. Soften the butter in a skillet over moderate heat. As soon as it has melted, whisk in the honey and bring to a boil. Decrease heat and simmer for 2 minutes.

2. Include apples and sauté for 10 minutes, or until the apples are browned and soft.

3. Blend in coconut milk and sea salt and bring to a boil once more. Decrease temperature and simmer for 5 minutes.

4. Take away from the heat and place at room temperature for 10-15 minutes to allow the syrup to thicken.

4.5. Chocolate Strawberry Waffles

Yield: 1-2 waffles

Ingredients

3 tbsp. chocolate protein powder
1 tbsp. ground flax seed
1 ½ tbsp. tapioca starch/flour
1 tbsp. unsweetened cocoa powder
¼ tsp. baking soda
½ tsp. vanilla extract
2-3 tbsp. almond milk
3 tbsp. liquid egg whites or 1 egg
¼ cup finely chopped strawberries
More chopped strawberries, nut butter, nuts, etc. for garnish (also optional)

1. Include protein powder, flax seed, tapioca starch, cocoa powder, baking soda, and stevia (if using) in a bowl and whisk to intermix.

2. Put in vanilla extract, egg whites or egg, and almond milk in a different bowl and whisk to mix.

3. Include wet ingredients to the dry ingredients and merge. Your batter will be similar to a smooth brownie batter. If this seems too thick, include a bit more almond milk or egg whites. If too runny, add additional protein powder.

4. Include your strawberries.

5. Warm up your waffle iron and grease with coconut oil.

6. As soon as waffle iron is prepared, apply about a heaping ¼ cup to measure out the batter and put onto the waffle iron, spreading it out a little bit. (It will eventually spread out during the cooking process)

7. Close up the waffle maker and wait.

8. The waffle should be done after approximately 3-5 minutes, dependent on the waffle maker.

9. Replicate with the left over batter

10. Top with additional chopped strawberries if preferred, and if you happen to be a huge chocolate lover, melt some Raw Mio.

5. Breakfast Sausages And Meat Recipes

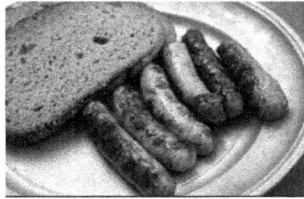

5.1. Chicken And Apple Sausage

Yield: 4 servings

Ingredients

2 large chicken breasts, or use 1 lb. ground chicken
1 apple, peeled and finely diced
1 Tablespoon fresh thyme leaves, finely chopped (or use 2 Tablespoons dried thyme)
3 Tablespoons fresh parsley, finely chopped
1 Tablespoon fresh oregano, finely chopped (or use 2 Tablespoons dried oregano)
2 teaspoons garlic powder
Salt and pepper
Coconut oil to cook with

Instructions

1. Pre-heat stove to 425F.

2. Place 3 tablespoons of coconut oil into a pan and cook (on a medium-high temperature) the apples, thyme, parsley, and oregano until the apples soften (7-8 minutes).

3. Take away from heat and let cool off for 5 minutes.

4. Food process the chicken breast (if you're not utilizing ground chicken meat).

5. Blend the chicken meat with everything in the pan, along with the garlic powder, salt and pepper (as well as any leftover oil).

6. Shape 12 thin patties (1/2 inch thick) from the meat and position on a baking tray lined with aluminum foil.

7. Bake for 20 minutes. Confirm with a meat thermometer that the interior temperature of a patty near the center of the tray is 170F.

8. Cool down and store in fridge or freezer (reheat easily in the mornings in the pan or in the microwave).

9. If you desire the sausages to be browned, then simply pan-fry for a couple of minutes in coconut oil. You may also pan-fry the raw sausages rather than putting them into the oven.

5.2. Breakfast Turkey Pear Patties

Yield: 10 servings

Instructions

1 lb. ground turkey
1 ripe pear, peeled and chopped
2 cloves garlic, minced
1 teaspoon fresh ginger, grated

1 teaspoon fresh sage, minced
1 teaspoon fresh rosemary, minced
1 teaspoon sea salt
1/2 teaspoon black pepper
1-2 tablespoons coconut oil

1. Beat pear in a food processor until it is smoothed out. In a mid-size bowl, mix turkey, pear, garlic, ginger, sage, rosemary, salt and pepper.

2. Form mix into small patties by rolling them into a ball in the palm of your hand and flattening them.

3. Heat up 1 tablespoon of coconut oil in a large bottomed pan, similar to cast iron. Include enough patties, so that they are not packed in the pan. You will need to cook these in two batches.

4. Cook for 4-5 minutes on the first side, until slightly browned and the patty raises from the pan easily.

5. Turnover and cook them on the second side for 2 to 3 minutes, or until they are surely browned on both sides and no longer pink inside. Shift cooked patties to a plate and set aside.

6. Add coconut oil if needed and cook the second batch of patties. Enjoy!

5.3. Apple Chutney Turkey Meatballs

Yield: 10 servings

Ingredients

Meatballs
1 lb. ground turkey (preferably the fattier grind or you may need to add a few tablespoons of oil)
1/2 teaspoon granulated garlic
1 teaspoon dehydrated onion flakes
1 teaspoon garam masala
1 teaspoon salt

Apple Chutney
3 medium (tart) apples, diced
1/2 handful raisins
2 tablespoons butter
1/2 teaspoon garam masala
3 tablespoons maple syrup
2 tablespoons mango chutney (optional)
1 tablespoon apple cider vinegar
1/4 cup water
1/4 teaspoon salt

Instructions

1. Pre-heat your oven to 400ºF.

2. Line a baking sheet with parchment paper or a silicone mat.

3. In a sizable bowl, intermix all of the turkey meatball ingredients. Make use of your hands, or a cookie scoop, to section into balls.

4. Bake until the meatballs are cooked all the way through, approximately 15-20 minutes, determined by the size.

Apple Chutney

1. Combine all of the ingredients into a mid-size sauce pot.

2. Cover up with a lid, slightly ajar, and stir frequently, over medium-high temperature, until the apples have softened, approximately 6-8 minutes.

3. Take away the lid and allow some of the liquid evaporate and decrease (if it hasn't already). Taste and adjust for seasoning.

4. Work with a tater masher to mash up the apples into a chunky chutney—not applesauce, but yet like 3/4 chunky, 1/4 smooth.
 Note: Use the chutney like a condiment for the meatballs—it's not a side dish.

5.4. Bacon Breakfast Sausage

Yield: 10-14 servings

Ingredients

4-5 thick-cut strips of smoked bacon
3/4 cup chopped leeks (white ends)
1 medium apple, cored and quartered (no need to peel, if organic)
1 tablespoon fresh or dried rosemary
2 tablespoon fresh chopped sage leaves (or 2 tsp of dried)
1 tablespoon molasses (honey would work too, just use a bit less)
1/2 tablespoon fresh lemon juice or apple cider vinegar

1/2 teaspoon ground black pepper
1 – 2 teaspoons sea salt, depending on personal taste
1/4 teaspoon ground cloves
A dash of cayenne powder
1 kilo or 2 lbs. ground pork

1. Bake the strips of bacon on a baking sheet at 400º F for a couple of minutes , until the rashers are nearly half-way done– this will take out some of the moisture , along with a small amount of the grease .

2. Place all of the ingredients aside from the pork into your food processor, and whiz until things are pretty finely chopped. You may have to scrape down the sides a couple of times, so that you don't have virtually any long strands of leeks.

3 .Once it's all equally chopped up, include the ground pork, and simply pulse for a few seconds until it looks as though it's all blended well– if you go too long, it makes the consistency too crumbly.

4. Season to desire taste. Whenever you're ready, shape them into little patties, and lay them out on a sizable baking sheet.

5. It is possible to flash-freeze these for a few hours, take the frozen patties from the baking sheet and store them. Whenever you're ready for an excellent breakfast, simply pull some from the freezer and prepare them in a lightly oiled skillet. You may also bake them in the oven at 350º F for 30 minutes– a terrific way to prepare a large amount of them for breakfast!

5.5. Spicy Italian Sausage Stuffed Peppers

Yield: 3-5 servings

Instructions

1 pound of ground Italian hot sausage.
5 assorted bell peppers. I went with 2 green, 2 red, 1 yellow.
1/2 head of cauliflower, grated or chopped into a "rice" consistency.
1 small (8 ounce) can of tomato paste.
1 small white onion, medium dice.
1/2 head of garlic, minced.
1 small handful of fresh basil, minced (or 2 tsp. dried).
2 tsp dried oregano.
2 tsp dried thyme.

Instructions

1. Chop the tops from your peppers and scoop out and throw out the seed, reserve the tops.

2. Process or cut approximately half a head of cauliflower into "rice" and add in a big mixing bowl.

3. Combine your minced garlic, basil, and dried herbs, and onion to your cauliflower and blend by hand.

4. Utilize a very hot skillet to slightly brown your sausage. The sausage will probably cook just fine in your slow cooker, however I personally prefer to hit it with a bit of sear to take the taste up a notch.

5. Include your sausage and a can of tomato paste to your bowl of seasoned cauliflower and combine by hand.

6. Fit as much of your sausage mix into your peppers as possible.

7. Position your peppers into the slow cooker and loosely position the pepper tops back on. If in case you have additional meat and cauliflower mixture, simply jam in the middle of your peppers and allow it to cook.

8. Cook on low heat for 6 hours.

6. Breakfast Wraps And Tortillas

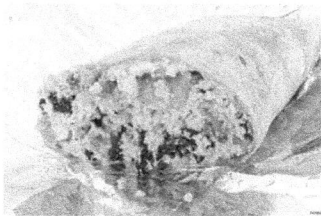

6.1. Cabbage, Bacon, Avocado Burrito W/ Sweet Potato Noddles

Yield: 2 servings

Ingredients

2 cabbage savoy leafs
1 avocado, insides cubed
Salt and pepper, to taste
4 pieces of bacon
1 sweet potato, peeled, Blade C
4 eggs, beaten

Instructions

1. Cleanse your cabbage leaves and pat dry. Reserve, on a plate.

2. Position your avocado into a bowl, mash and season with salt and pepper. Spread this over the middle of every cabbage leaf.

3. Place a sizable skillet over moderate heat and add the bacon. Allow it to cook until to your crispy preference and put aside on a paper-towel lined plate.

4. Take away half of the oil left behind from the bacon and put in your sweet potato noodles. Cook the noodles, tossing frequently, for 5-8 minutes or until they wilt. As soon as they are done, place onto the cabbage leaves, over the avocado.

5. Then, set the eggs into the same skillet and scramble. When scrambled, set over the sweet potato noodles.

6. Top the eggs with 2 pieces of bacon per wrap. And then, roll like a burrito and enjoy.

6.2. Breakfast Egg Burrito

Yield: 2 servings

Instructions

4 eggs, whites and yolks separated
1/2 onion, finely chopped
1 to 2 tomatoes, finely chopped
1/4 cup canned diced green chilies
1 red pepper, cut into strips
1/4 cup finely chopped cilantro
1/2 cup cooked meat (try sliced steak, ground beef, or shredded chicken)
1 avocado, cut into wedges or small chunks
Hot sauce or salsa on the side

Instructions

1. Whisk the egg whites

2. Heat a lightly oiled 10-inch skillet. Pour half the egg whites in the pan, swirling the pan around so the whites stretch thinly and evenly.

3. After approximately 30 seconds, place a lid on the pan and cook 1 minute extra. Make use of a rubber spatula to release and slide the egg white "tortilla" onto a dish or plate.

4. Replicate once again with the left over egg whites.

5. In the same pan, sauté onions with oil for 1 minute then insert tomato, green chills, red pepper, cilantro, and meat.

6. Whisk egg yolks and fill into the pan, blending into a scramble with the other ingredients.

7. Insert avocado at the very end, and then spoon half of filling onto each egg white.

8. Roll the egg whites up into burritos and serve up with hot sauce or salsa.

6.3. Guacamole Topped Breakfast Quesadillas

Yield: 1-2 serving

Ingredients

2 grain free flax tortilla wraps
1 tsp ghee or coconut oil
3 large organic eggs + 1 tsp ghee
Handful of spinach chopped
Pinch of Himalayan Rock Salt and Black Pepper
2 tbsp. homemade harissa plus more for topping

Quick Guacamole
1/2 a large ripe avocado mashed
Dash of lime juice
Salt and pepper to taste
Coriander and Lime wedges to serve

1. Whisk collectively eggs with salt and pepper.

2. Put in a pot with melted ghee over a low to moderate heat. Whisk after one minute to break up the curds. Cook for 1 to 2 minutes more; take away from the heat while still not completely set!

3. Mix through chopped spinach.

4. Spread every tortilla with a tbsp. of the harissa on one side. Set half the egg mix in to each and fold over.

5. Place into a hot pan with melted ghee and cook every one, for 2-3 minute per side or until lightly browned and crisp.

6. Serve up immediately divided in half. Top with quick guacamole and a little additional dollop of harissa on top.

6.4. Bacon Avocado Egg Salad Wraps

Yield: 1-2 servings

Ingredients

1 ripe avocado
Juice of 1/2 lemon
4 hard-boiled eggs, chilled
2 Tablespoons celery
1 Tablespoon chopped parsley
1/2 teaspoon salt
1/4 teaspoon freshly ground pepper
1 head butter crunch lettuce
4-5 endive bulbs
1-2 slices of cooked bacon

Instructions

1. In a mid-size bowl, mash avocado and fresh lemon juice together with a fork until it is creamy and smoothed out. It is alright if there are still a couple of lumps.

2. With a box grater over the bowl, grate in the 4 hard-boiled eggs. Include the chopped celery, parsley, and seasonings to the bowl.

3. Blend gradually with a fork until everything is combined. Taste the egg salad and modify the seasonings as needed.

4. At this time the mix can be refrigerated for approximately 2 hours.

5. Break off the lettuce or endive leaves and organize them on a plate.

6. Spoon the egg salad into the lettuce cups and top with chopped bacon and parsley. Serve immediately.

6.5. Vegetable And Egg White Wrap

Yield: 4 servings

Ingredients

3 Egg whites
Handful of spinach
7 Cherry tomatoes (halved)
½ cup Frozen onions and;
Bell pepper mix
Coconut oil to grease pan
Garlic powder
Sea salt
Ground pepper

Ingredients

1. Making use of a mixer or hand mixer, whisk the egg whites and seasonings for 1 minute.

2. In sizable pan warmed up to medium and greased, cook egg whites and cover up with lid. Make sure to work with a large level pan so the eggs can spread out thinly and evenly.

3. Be careful not to flip the eggs, so make sure that the heat is low enough that it won't burn up the eggs before they are completely cooked through.

4. When egg wrap is cooking, microwave the frozen vegetables for 1 minute and dice the cherry tomatoes in halves.

5. When the egg is cooked, transfer from pan onto plate or dish. It should slide off the pan.

6. Sauté the spinach, onions, bell peppers, and tomatoes on medium-high temperature. I cook them until I start to see slight browning on the tomatoes.

7. Gradually add sautéed vegetables to the wrap, and cover the egg around the top like you would for a tortilla wrap.

8. The wrap is delicate, so eat it with a fork.

Part 2

Introduction To Paleo Diet

The Paleo diet also called as caveman diet. This Diet is based mainly on foods presumed to have been available to Stone-Age man. The Paleo diet is about consuming food which existing since Paleolithic period

The Paleolithic period was pre-agricultural period. In Paleo diet the technique of consuming food goes back to fundamental way of eating. Paleolithic diets are about consuming food the way our predecessors did.

The Paleo diet is primarily focused authentic foods which have been consumed for thousands of years. Paleo diet followers should eat as organically as possible like grass-fed meats, fruit, vegetables, nuts and seeds

This way of diet eliminates the artificial foods, salt, sugar additives, and highly processed foods. Paleo diet helps to progressing from consuming processed foods to whole foods it is practically unfeasible not to make improved eating choices and start feeling healthier

The Paleo diet is quite low in carbohydrates, but loaded in high protein and healthy fats, which help the body to add fibre, vitamins and minerals. The Paleo diet does not encourage cold cut meats yet allows to consume fruits and vegetables that have alkaline in them

The diet is not low in fat but instead it adds addition of natural fats from grass fed cattle, fish, seafood, nuts, seeds and oils. The abolition of such an extensive assortment of foods, such as grains, dairy, processed foods and sugar implies the diet is possible to lead to significant weight loss

The greatest features of the Paleo diet is, it can be tailored to your exact health requirements or conditions, such as food allergy, religious practices, or moral restraints.

The Benefits of Paleo Diet

1. Weight Loss

The Paleo diet is a low carbohydrate diet getting rid of junk and refined food will radically cut carbohydrate which results in weight loss. By restricting carbohydrates intake, Paleo helps to eliminate unnecessary weight gain. Paleo plays a major part in reducing waist lines and stubborn fat by burning excess fat

2. Better Digestion and Absorption

Eating of food that has adapted over thousands of years ago. This means that food was consumed in its simplest form and therefore was easy on digestion. If digestive problems are recurring, trying Paleo diet for at least a month will make you feel healthier for sure.

3. Provide Vitamins & Minerals

The Paleo diet advocates consuming the "rainbow", the diverse colors of vegetables. Vegetables are a great component of the Vitamins. Eating vegetables and fruits is the best way to stock up on the essential nutrients. The diverse colors of vegetables indicate the presence of a variety of nutrients

4. Enhance Brain Function

The supplies of protein and fat recommended by the Paleo diet emerges from wild salmon. Salmon is full of omega 3 fatty acids which is deficient in the standard diet. Since omega 3 fatty acids have DHA, acknowledged to be excellent for eyes, heart, and improvement brain and multi-tasking

5. Fewer Allergies

The Paleo diet eliminate allergic foods. Food which are unable to digest like seeds, grains, and dairy which is the reason for which the Paleo diet advocates the elimination of these food products, when most diets do not skip these food, and the people affected are considerably in control of their allergies after the Paleo regime

6. Improve Health

Sugar, salt, artificial fats, and other refined edibles cause inflammation inside the intestinal tract. Sadly, when unnecessary amount of processed foods met with a lot of anxiety, the result the intestinal walls are infringed and things that do not generally leave the passage end up seeping out

Clearly a person wants to keep the fare in the digestive tract until it is all set to be brought to your cells, so that energy can be produced.

Eating Paleo can help indefinitely with the problem, because processed food and sugars are eliminated, leaving little to no chance of a mishap occurring.

7. Healthy Cells

Each cell in the body is made with a combination of saturated and unsaturated fat. The Paleo diet offers an ideal equilibrium of fats, since both saturated and unsaturated fats exist in adequate quantities in the Paleo diet, while other diets lack one or the other fat

8. Reduce Inflammation

Studies show that inflammation is the primary issue behind cardiovascular disease. The Paleo diet focuses solely on food items that are anti-inflammatory, thereby reducing the risk of heart disease significantly. The presence of omega 3 fatty acids is one of the reasons for which the Paleo diet is anti-inflammatory

9. New Energy

Breakfast cereals and any food that are advertised to give energy really drain you of it. When following the Paleo diet, there has been reported significant increase in energy due to the high protein content

10 Increased Insulin Sensitivity

When a person regularly supplies their body with sugary and junk food, in time the body numbs itself to the food as it does not desire or require them. This is where the surplus sugar and carbohydrates store up, because they do not have a specific use for their energy, the cells reject them. This leads to insulin sensitivity where the body will be inept in identifying when the cells are filled or not

How Paleo Helps to Lose Weight?

The paleo diet converts the body from a principally carbohydrate-burning machine into a fat-burning machine. This is the reason why many find that Paleo diet to be a successful way for losing weight. This is because the human body almost derives its ideal source of energy from fats

Fat takes a lot of time to be burned and it is more resourceful for the body. But as soon as we acquire extra carbohydrates more than what is required for our energy use, the body store the rest as fat for later, in case starvation is on the horizon. Fortunately, a large amount of people will in no way be in risk of starvation.

Hence, a person has no means of using the stored fat meant for emergencies for energy; so instead of burning the fat that has already been stored up in the body, people just keep piling more over again

This is the key reason for majority of western countries have an obesity epidemic. The Paleo diet revolutionizes this problem with one simple strategy: eliminate plain carbohydrates from everyday meals

Mainly, it simply means that by cutting down the quantity of carbohydrate intake, the Paleo diet permits the body to initiate the route of burning fat, hence leading to prominent weight loss

What Can We Eat on a Paleo Diet?

The Paleo diet is more of a lifestyle change. Sometimes it helps to educate yourself about just how unhealthy processed foods can be for you. It can also help to start growing your own garden so you have access to nutritious fruits and vegetables that you helped to cultivate yourself. Not only is it easy on the wallet, but it's empowering.

The foods you are allowed to eat on a Paleo diet can be broken down to these basic essentials:

1. Vegetables

An unfortunate aspect of the SAD diet is how it treats fruits and vegetables. Only a few vegetables are commonly eaten: potatoes, corn, and, every once in a while, broccoli. And usually these are lathered with butter and cheese.

The Paleo diet demands great utilization of vegetables, preferably as raw as possible to guarantee the ability to detoxify the body of toxins, including the BPA all too often consumed from canned vegetables and fruit.

2. Fruits

Fruits should be organic whenever possible to prevent consumption of pesticides into the body that can lead to disruptions in hormonal functions and other complications. Fruits are a good substitute for artificially sweetened snacks and desserts that are typically found in the SAD diet

3. Nuts

It is rare to stumble upon a person who eats enough nuts and seeds in their diet. Nuts can be a bit pricey, possibly because there is such a low demand for them, and many people suffer from nut allergies.

However, they are full of proteins, healthy fats, and oils that were used by our ancestors to stay alert. They contribute to positive muscle growth and make a great snack when you're on the go.

4. Meat

Meat may be most people's favorite part of the Paleo diet. Meat is full of proteins that help build our muscles and maintain athleticism, and our ancestors often depended upon meat from a hunt for survival.

Stay away from factory farmed foods; the animals are treated cruelly and are served a cocktail of antibiotics and growth hormones that find their way into our bodies. As you can imagine, these are toxins that ultimately worsen our health and impede weight-loss and other positive results of the Paleo diet.

5. Seeds

Seeds offer great nutritional benefits, but because they are high in fat, it's possible for them to become rancid, so be careful not to buy more than you can eat in a reasonable amount of time and store them in dark, cool places with low humidity.

If the seeds have already been removed from their hulls they will expire faster. Seeds are full of great things like iron (sometimes having even more than meat!), calcium, niacin, fiber, and folic-acid.

What Not to Eat When Going Paleo

Every diet ends up with restrictions. In the case of the Paleo diet, there are a few things you'll want to stay away from.

- Processed/boxed foods
- Canned fruits and vegetables.
- Most dairy products (They are full of growth hormones)
- Anything with artificial ingredients. (nitrates, MSG, calcium sorbate, aspartame, artificial colors, saccharin, sorbic acid, potassium bromate, any and all GMOs, and all artificial sweeteners)
- Oils full of trans fats or partly hydrogenated oils.
- Fast food
- High Fructose Corn Syrup. (in most junk foods)
- Legumes (phytic acid)
- Grains and pseudograins. (phytic acid)
- Potatoes
- Soda

Our ancestors survived just fine without most of these things. Although many were present during the time of the caveman and used for survival, in order to maintain a Paleo diet that not only provides us with great health but also helps us to lose weight and maintain lean muscle, we will need to make a few sacrifices

Types of Paleo Diets

One of the greatest features of the Paleo diet is that it can be tailored to your exact health requirements or conditions, such as food allergy, religious practices, or moral restraints.

There are many types of paleo but here we focus on three widely followed types of paleo diet.

1. The Basic Paleo

This is the standard Paleo diet rejects grains, dairy, soy, refined and processed foods. It also omits bogus fats, in addition to vegetable oils that are excessively processed.

2. The Ketogenic Paleo

The most vital in low-carbohydrate, the ketogenic diet makes the body into a state of ketosis where fat is the main fuel as an alternative of glucose. Ketogenic consumption can be prepared inside the restrictions of a Paleo regimen.

Ketogenic Paleo is mainly consumed by those who have a great amount of weight to lose, diabetics, or body builders. It can, moreover, be made use of to keep up a wellness arrangement for epilepsy.

3. The 80/ 20 Paleo

When Paleo was originally growing to be accepted, some supporters advised being Paleo 80% of the time, while saving the remaining 20% for non-Paleo foods.

This can be taken up by people who are in the Paleo lifestyle as they are a family unit, or persons who have by now accomplished their physical condition targets.

Getting Started

Paleo diet is not like other classical diets. You need to open your mind and widen your understanding of what Paleolithic diet really means and how you will advance in it

Paleo diet is not about calculating calories, carbohydrates, or fat. The diet works not because of calorie counting but for the body is getting rid of stored up fat, along with a lot of harmful things that would eventually be a threat.

There are two types of Paleolithic followers:

1. Classic Followers:

These type of Paleo followers go accurately. They will not permit grains of any category, refined sugar, everything dairy, will look for pasture-fed meats and natural fruits and vegetables, consume freshly caught game, and aspire to pursue the set of rules word for word

2. Modern Followers:

These type of Paleo followers take a laidback approach, and understand that in the current world it is not realistic to eat precisely like a caveman, and they include some contemporary comfort into their Paleo style.

They may add little dairy every so often, or be happy with pseudo-grains, or even include a non-Paleo meal per month. Regardless of which way one chooses the Paleo diet will work, as you simply follow its basic principles. One does consume much better food, cutting oneself off from the fast food that surrounds us each day

1. In Early Weeks:

In early weeks of Paleo can be little tough, mainly for those who don't try any kind of diet earlier

Purging sugar from the system can be tough for individuals who have consumed a diet loaded with sugary substances. Eliminating bread and other grain-based food can also be rough. The early various person to person but it is typically 4 to 8 weeks

2. After Early Weeks:

After early weeks, your path will not be rocky anymore. The diet starts working; you begin to drop weight until you attain a physically healthy weight. You have more energy than in the past. This is wonderful comes alive

Breakfast Recipes

Coconut And Almonds Granola

(**Prep + Cook Time**: 45 minutes | **Servings**: 4)

Ingredients:

- 3 cups coconut flakes
- 1½ cups almonds; chopped
- 1/2 cup sesame seeds
- 1/2 cup sunflower seeds

- 1/2 tsp. cinnamon; ground
- 2 tbsp. chia seeds
- 1/2 cup maple syrup
- A pinch of cardamom
- 1 tsp. vanilla extract
- 2 tbsp. olive oil

Instructions:
1. In a bowl; mix almonds with sunflower seeds, sesame seeds, coconut, chia seeds, cardamom and cinnamon and stir.
2. Meanwhile; heat up a small pot over medium heat, add oil, vanilla and maple syrup, stir well and cook for about 1 minute.
3. Pour this over almonds mix, stir everything, spread on a baking sheet, bake in the oven at 300 °F for 25 minutes, stirring the mixture after 15 minutes. Leave your special granola to cool down before dividing it between plates and serving it.

Nutrition Facts Per Serving: Calories: 270; Fat: 13; Fiber: 5; Carbs: 7; Protein: 8

Tomato And Eggs Breakfast

(**Prep + Cook Time**: 40 minutes | **Servings**: 2)

Ingredients:
- 2 tomatoes
- 2 eggs
- A pinch of black pepper
- 1 tsp. parsley; finely chopped

Instructions:
1. Cut tomatoes tops, scoop flesh and arrange them on a lined baking sheet.
2. Crack an egg in each tomato.
3. Season with salt and pepper. Introduce them in the oven at 350 °F and bake for 30 minutes.

4. Take tomatoes out of the oven, divide between plates, season with pepper, sprinkle parsley at the end and serve.

Nutrition Facts Per Serving: Calories: 186; Protein: 14; Fat: 10; Sugar: 6

Plantain Pancakes

(**Prep + Cook Time**: 20 minutes | **Servings**: 1)

Ingredients:
- 1/2 plantain; peeled and chopped
- 1 tbsp. shaved coconut; toasted for serving
- 1 tbsp. coconut milk for serving
- 3 eggs
- 1/4 cup coconut flour
- 1/4 cup coconut water
- 1 tsp. coconut oil
- 1/4 tsp. cream of tartar
- 1/4 tsp. baking soda
- 1/4 tsp. chai spice

Instructions:
1. In your food processor, mix eggs with coconut water and flour, plantain, cream of tartar, baking soda and chai spice and blend well.
2. Heat up a pan with the coconut oil over medium heat, add 1/4 cup pancake batter, spread evenly, cook until it becomes golden, flip pancake and cook for 1 more minute and transfer to a plate.
3. Repeat this with the rest of the batter. Serve pancakes with shaved coconut and coconut milk.

Nutrition Facts Per Serving: Calories: 372; Fat: 17; Carbs: 55; Fiber: 12; Sugar: 21; Protein: 23

Muffins Breakfast

(**Prep + Cook Time**: 40 minutes | **Servings**: 4)

Ingredients:

- 1 cup kale; chopped
- Some coconut oil for greasing the muffin cups
- 1/4 cup chives; finely chopped
- 1/2 cup almond milk
- 6 eggs
- Black pepper to the taste

Instructions:
1. In a bowl; mix eggs with chives and kale and whisk very well.
2. Add black pepper to the taste and almond milk and stir well.
3. Divide this into 8 muffin cups after you've greased it with some coconut oil.
4. Introduce this in preheated oven at 350 °F and bake for 30 minutes. Take muffins out of the oven, leave them to cool down, transfer them to plates and serve warm.

Nutrition Facts Per Serving: Calories: 100; Fat: 5; Protein: 14; Sugar: 0

Paleo Pork Skillet

(**Prep + Cook Time**: 30 minutes | **Servings**: 4)
Ingredients:
- 8 oz. mushrooms; chopped
- 1 lb. pork; ground
- 1 tbsp. olive oil
- Black pepper to the taste
- 2 zucchinis; cut in halves and then in half moons
- 1/2 tsp. garlic powder
- 1/2 tsp. basil; dried
- A pinch of sea salt
- 2 tbsp. Dijon mustard

Instructions:
1. Heat up a pan with the oil over medium high heat, add mushrooms, stir and cook for 4 minutes.

2. Add zucchinis, a pinch of salt and black pepper, stir and cook for 4 minutes more.
3. Add pork, garlic powder and basil, stir and cook until meat is done. Add mustard, stir well, cook for a couple more minutes, divide between plates and serve.

Nutrition Facts Per Serving: Calories: 200; Fat: 4; Fiber: 2; Carbs: 5; Protein: 12

Squash Blossom Frittata

(**Prep + Cook Time**: 50 minutes | **Servings**: 4)

Ingredients:
- 10 eggs; whisked
- Black pepper to the taste
- 1/4 cup coconut cream
- 1 yellow onion; finely chopped
- 1 leek; thinly sliced
- 2 scallions; thinly sliced
- 2 zucchinis; chopped
- 8 squash blossoms
- 2 tbsp. avocado oil

Instructions:
1. In a bowl; mix eggs with coconut cream and black pepper to the taste and stir well.
2. Heat up a pan with the oil over medium high heat, add leek and onions, stir and cook for 5 minutes.
3. Add zucchini, stir and cook for 10 more minutes.
4. Add eggs, spread, reduce heat to low, cook for 5 minutes.
5. Sprinkle scallions and arrange squash blossoms on frittata, press blossoms into eggs, introduce everything in the oven at 350 °F and bake for 20 minutes. Take frittata out of the oven, leave it to cool down, cut, arrange on plates and serve it.

Nutrition Facts Per Serving: Calories: 123; Fat: 8; Protein: 7; Carbs: 2; Sugar: 0

Turkey Breakfast Sandwich

(Prep + Cook Time: 5 minutes | **Servings**: 1)

Ingredients:

- 2 oz. turkey meat; roasted and thinly sliced
- 2 tbsp. pecans; toasted and chopped
- 2 slices paleo coconut bread
- 2 tbsp. cranberry chutney
- 1/4 cup arugula

Instructions:

1. In a bowl; mix pecans with chutney and stir well.
2. Spread this on bread slice, add turkey slices and arugula and top with the other bread slice. Serve right away.

Nutrition Facts Per Serving: Calories: 540; Fat: 11; Carbs: 52; Fiber: 4; Sugar: 13; Protein: 32

Sweet Potato Paleo Breakfast

(Prep + Cook Time: 25 minutes | **Servings**: 4)

Ingredients:

- 2 Italian sausages; casings removed
- 4 tbsp. coconut oil
- 1 small green bell pepper; chopped
- 1/2 cup onion; chopped
- 2 garlic cloves; minced
- 2 cups sweet potato; chopped
- 1 avocado; peeled, pitted, cut into halves and thinly sliced
- 3 eggs
- 2 cups spinach

Instructions:

1. Heat up a pan with the oil over medium high heat, add onion, stir and cook for 3 minutes.
2. Add garlic and bell pepper, stir and cook for 1 minute.
3. Add sausage meat, stir and brown for 4 minutes more.
4. Add sweet potato, stir and cook for 4 minutes.

5. Add spinach, stir and cook for 2 minutes.
6. Make 3 holes in this mix, crack an egg in each, introduce pan in preheated broiler and cook for 3 minutes. Divide this tasty mix on plates, add avocado pieces on the side and serve.

Nutrition Facts Per Serving: Calories: 200; Fat: 4; Fiber: 2; Carbs: 6; Protein: 9

Homemade Breakfast Granola

(**Prep + Cook Time**: 55 minutes | **Servings**: 6)

Ingredients:
- 2 tsp. cinnamon powder
- 1½ cups almond flour
- 2 tsp. nutmeg; ground
- 1/2 cup coconut flakes
- 2 tsp. vanilla extract
- 1/2 cup walnuts; chopped
- 1/3 cup coconut oil
- 1/4 cup hemp hearts

Instructions:
1. In a bowl; combine almond flour with coconut flakes, walnuts, cinnamon, nutmeg, vanilla, hemp and walnuts, stir well and spread on a baking sheet.
2. Bake in the oven at 275 °F and bake for 50 minutes, stirring every 10 minutes. Transfer to plates when the granola is cold and serve for breakfast.

Nutrition Facts Per Serving: Calories: 250; Fat: 23; Fiber: 4; Carbs: 5; Protein: 6

Italian Style Eggs

(**Prep + Cook Time**: 25 minutes | **Servings**: 1)

Ingredients:
- 2 eggs
- 1/4 tsp. rosemary; dried
- 1/2 cup cherry tomatoes halved

- 1½ cups kale; chopped
- 1/2 tsp. coconut oil
- 3 tbsp. water
- 1 tsp. balsamic vinegar
- 1/4 avocado; peeled and chopped

Instructions:

1. Heat up a pan with the oil over medium high heat, add water, kale, rosemary and tomatoes, stir; cover and cook for 4 minutes.
2. Uncover pan, stir again and add eggs.
3. Stir and scramble eggs for 3 minutes.
4. Add vinegar, stir everything and transfer to a serving plate. Top with chopped avocado and serve.

Nutrition Facts Per Serving: Calories: 185; Fat: 10; Fiber: 1; Carbs: 6; Protein: 7

Red Breakfast Smoothie

(**Prep + Cook Time**: 5 minutes | **Servings**: 2)

Ingredients:

- 1 small red bell pepper; seeded and roughly chopped
- 5 strawberries; cut in halves
- 1 tomato; cut into 4 wedges
- 1 cup red cabbage; chopped
- 1/2 cup raspberries
- 8 oz. water
- 2 ice cubes for serving

Instructions:

1. In your food processor, mix cabbage with bell pepper, tomato, strawberries and raspberries and pulse well until you obtain cream.
2. Add water and pulse well a few more times. Transfer to glasses and serve with ice cubes.

Nutrition Facts Per Serving: Calories: 189; Fat: 2; Carbs: 40; Fiber: 7; Sugar: 1; Protein: 5

Maple Nut Porridge

(**Prep + Cook Time**: 10 minutes | **Servings**: 2)

Ingredients:
- 2 tbsp. coconut butter
- 1/2 cup pecans; soaked
- 3/4 cup hot water
- 1 banana; peeled and chopped
- 1/2 tsp. cinnamon
- 2 tsp. maple syrup

Instructions:
1. In your food processor, mix pecans with water, coconut butter, banana, cinnamon and maple syrup and blend well.
2. Transfer this to a pan, heat up over medium heat until it thickens, pour into bowls and serve.

Nutrition Facts Per Serving: Calories: 170; Fat: 9; Carbs: 20; Fiber: 6; Protein: 6

Tasty Nuts Porridge

(**Prep + Cook Time**: 15 minutes | **Servings**: 2)

Ingredients:
- 1/2 cup pecans; soaked overnight and drained
- 1/2 banana; mashed
- 3/4 cup hot water
- 2 tbsp. coconut butter
- 1/2 tsp. cinnamon
- 2 tsp. maple syrup

Instructions:
1. In a blender, mix pecans, with water, banana, coconut butter, cinnamon and maple syrup, pulse really well and transfer to a small pot.

2. Heat everything up over medium heat, cook until it's creamy, transfer to serving bowls and serve.

Nutrition Facts Per Serving: Calories: 150; Fat: 2; Fiber: 2; Carbs: 4; Protein: 6

Eggs And Artichokes

(**Prep + Cook Time**: 50 minutes | **Servings**: 2)

Ingredients:
- 1 egg white
- 4 whole eggs
- 3/4 cup balsamic vinegar
- 4 oz. bacon; chopped
- 4 artichoke hearts
- A pinch of sea salt
- Black pepper to the taste

For the sauce:
- 1 tbsp. lemon juice
- 3/4 cup ghee
- 4 egg yolks
- A pinch of paprika

Instructions:
1. Put artichoke hearts in a bowl; add vinegar, toss a bit and leave aside for 20 minutes.
2. Put the ghee in a pan and melt it over medium high heat.
3. In a bowl; mix 4 egg yolks with paprika and lemon juice and stir well. Put some water into a pot and bring to a simmer over medium heat.
4. Put the bowl with the egg yolks on top of simmering water and stir constantly.
5. Add melted ghee gradually, stir until sauce thickens and take off heat.
6. Drain artichokes, place them on a lined baking sheet, brush tops with 1 egg white, add bacon on top and season with black pepper and a pinch of sea salt.

7. Introduce them in the oven at 375 °F and bake for 20 minutes.
8. Meanwhile; heat up a pot with water and bring to a simmer over medium high heat.
9. Crack 4 eggs into simmering water but make sure you only crack one at a time.
10. Poach eggs for 1 minute and transfer them to plates. Add artichokes and bacon on the side, drizzle the sauce you've made earlier on top and served.

Nutrition Facts Per Serving: Calories: 270; Fat: 24; Fiber: 0; Carbs: 5; Protein: 16

Green Smoothie

(**Prep + Cook Time**: 5 minutes | **Servings**: 3)
Ingredients:
- 1 small cucumber; peeled and chopped
- 1 green apple; chopped
- Juice of 1/2 lemon
- Juice of 1/2 lime
- 1 tbsp. ginger; finely grated
- 1 tbsp. gelatin powder
- 1 cup kale; chopped
- 1 cup coconut water

Instructions:
1. In your kitchen blender, mix the apple with cucumber, ginger and kale and pulse a few times.
2. Add lime and lemon juice, coconut water and gelatin powder and blend a few more times. Transfer to glasses and serve right away.

Nutrition Facts Per Serving: Calories: 180; Fat: 1; Carbs: 42; Fiber: 7; Sugar: 0, protein7

Parsley And Pear Smoothie

(**Prep + Cook Time**: 5 minutes | **Servings**: 6)

Ingredients:
- 1 apple pear; chopped
- 1 bunch parsley; roughly chopped
- 1 small avocado; stoned and peeled
- 1 pear; peeled and chopped
- 1 green apple; chopped
- 1 Granny Smith apple; chopped
- 6 bananas; peeled and roughly chopped
- 2 plums; stoned
- 1 cup ice
- 1 cup water

Instructions:
1. In your kitchen blender, mix parsley with avocado, apple pear, pear, green apple, Granny Smith apple, plums and bananas and blend very well.
2. Add ice and water and blend again very well. Transfer to tall glasses and serve right away.

Nutrition Facts Per Serving: Calories: 208; Carbs: 48; Fiber: 13; Fat: 3; Protein: 3; Sugar: 28

Delicious Eggs And Ham

(**Prep + Cook Time**: 25 minutes | **Servings**: 4)

Ingredients:
- 4 eggs
- 10 ham slices
- 4 tbsp. scallions
- A pinch of black pepper
- A pinch of sweet paprika
- 1 tbsp. melted ghee

Instructions:
1. Grease a muffin pan with melted ghee.

2. Divide ham slicesin each muffin mold to form your cups. In a bowl; mix eggs with scallions, pepper and paprika and whisk well.
3. Divide this mix on top of ham, introduce your ham cups in the oven at 400 °F and bake for 15 minutes. Leave cups to cool down before dividing on plates and serving.

Nutrition Facts Per Serving: Calories: 250; Fat: 10; Fiber: 3; Carbs: 6; Protein: 12

Orange And Dates Granola

(Prep + Cook Time: 25 minutes | **Servings**: 6)
Ingredients:
- 5 oz. dates; soaked in hot water
- 1/2 cup pumpkin seeds
- Juice from 1 orange
- Grated rind of 1/2 orange
- 1 cup desiccated coconut
- 1/2 cup silvered almonds
- 1/2 cup linseeds
- 1/2 cup sesame seeds
- Almond milk for serving

Instructions:
1. In a bowl; mix almonds with orange rind, orange juice, linseeds, coconut, pumpkin and sesame seeds and stir well.
2. Drain dates, add them to your food processor and blend well. Add this paste to almonds mix and stir well again.
3. Spread this on a lined baking sheet, introduce in the oven at 350 °F and bake for 15 minutes, stirring every 4 minutes.
4. Take granola out of the oven, leave aside to cool down a bit and then serve with almond milk.

Nutrition Facts Per Serving: Calories: 208; Protein: 6; Fiber: 5; Fat: 9; Sugar: 0

Blueberry Smoothie

(**Prep + Cook Time**: 5 minutes | **Servings**: 2)

Ingredients:

- 2 cups blueberries
- 1 tsp. lemon zest
- 1/2 cup coconut milk
- A pinch of cinnamon
- Water as needed

Instructions:

1. In your kitchen blender, mix coconut milk with blueberries, lemon zest and a pinch of cinnamon and pulse a few times.
2. Add water as needed to thin your smoothie and pulse a few more times. Transfer to a tall glass and serve.

Nutrition Facts Per Serving: Calories: 177; Fat: 3; Carbs: 45; Fiber: 7; Sugar: 12; Protein: 3

Paleo Cereal Bowl

(**Prep + Cook Time**: 10 minutes | **Servings**: 2)

Ingredients:

- 2 tbsp. pumpkin seeds
- 2 tbsp. almonds; chopped
- 1 tbsp. chia seeds
- A handful blueberries
- 1/3 cup water
- 1/3 cup almond milk

Instructions:

1. Put half of the pumpkin seeds in your food processor and blend them.
2. In 2 bowls, divide water, milk, the rest of the pumpkin seeds, chia seeds and almonds and stir.
3. Add blended pumpkin seeds and stir gently everything. Serve with blueberries on top.

Nutrition Facts Per Serving: Calories: 150; Fat: 3; Fiber: 4; Carbs: 5; Protein: 6

Delightful Sausage Balls

(Prep + Cook Time: 30 minutes | **Servings**: 8)

Ingredients:
- 2 eggs
- 1 tsp. baking soda
- 1 lb. sausage; chopped
- 1/4 cup coconut flour
- Black pepper to the taste
- 1 tsp. smoked paprika

Instructions:
1. In your food processor, mix sausage with eggs, baking soda, flour, pepper and paprika and pulse really well.
2. Shape medium balls from this mix, arrange them on a lined baking sheet and bake them in the oven at 350 °F for 20 minutes. Divide them between plates and serve in the morning.

Nutrition Facts Per Serving: Calories: 150; Fat: 7; Fiber: 3; Carbs: 4; Protein: 6

Breakfast Burger

(Prep + Cook Time: 30 minutes | **Servings**: 4)

Ingredients:
- 5 eggs
- 1 lb. ground beef meat
- 1/2 cup sausages; ground
- 8 slices bacon
- 3 sun-dried tomatoes; chopped
- 2 tbsp. almond meal
- 2 tsp. basil leaves; chopped
- 1 tsp. garlic; finely minced
- A drizzle of avocado oil
- Black pepper to the taste

Instructions:
1. In a bowl; mix beef meat with 1 egg, almond meal, tomatoes, basil, pepper and garlic, stir well and form 4 burgers.
2. Heat up a pan over medium high heat, add burgers, cook them 5 minutes on each side, transfer them to plates and leave aside for now.
3. Heat up the same pan over medium-high heat, add sausages, stir; cook for 5 minutes and transfer them to a plate.
4. Heat up the pan again, add bacon, cook for 4 minutes, drain excess grease and also leave aside on a plate.
5. Fry the 4 eggs in a pan with a drizzle of oil over medium-high heat and place them on top of burgers. ,Add sausage and bacon and serve.

Nutrition Facts Per Serving: Calories: 264; Fat: 12; Carbs: 5; Fiber: 0.3; Sugar: 0.7; Protein: 32

Simple Paleo Breakfast Waffles

(**Prep + Cook Time**: 20 minutes | **Servings**: 4)

Ingredients:
- 2 eggs
- 1/2 cup almond milk
- 2 tbsp. coconut oil; melted
- 1/2 tsp. cinnamon; ground
- 1 tbsp. baking powder
- 1 tbsp. coconut flour
- 2 tbsp. honey
- 1½ cups almond flour
- 1/4 cup tapioca flour
- 1½ tsp. vanilla extract
- Pure maple syrup for serving

Instructions:
1. In your mixer bowl; combine coconut flour with almond flour, tapioca flour, baking powder and cinnamon and stir.

2. Add egg yolks, almond milk, coconut oil, honey and vanilla extract and blend very well.
3. In another bowl; whisk egg whites with your mixer.
4. Add them to waffles mix and stir everything very well.
5. Pour this into your waffle iron and make 8 waffles. Divide them on plates, top with maple syrup and serve.

Nutrition Facts Per Serving: Calories: 160; Fat: 11; Fiber: 2; Carbs: 7; Protein: 6

Breakfast Pancakes

(Prep + Cook Time: 40 minutes | **Servings**: 4)

Ingredients:
- 12 bacon slices; chopped
- 8 eggs
- Black pepper to the taste
- 1½ tbsp. coconut oil
- 10 grain-free pancakes

For the pancakes:
- 1 cup arrowroot
- 1/2 cup almond flour
- 1/2 cup coconut flour
- 1/2 tsp. baking soda
- 1 tsp. cinnamon
- 1 cup almond milk
- 2 eggs
- 1 tsp. vanilla extract
- 3 tbsp. maple syrup
- 2 tbsp. coconut oil

Instructions:
1. In a bowl; mix arrowroot with almond flour, coconut flour, baking soda and cinnamon and stir.
2. Add almond milk, 2 eggs, vanilla extract and maple syrup and stir well until you obtain a smooth batter.

3. Heat up a pan with 2 tbsp. coconut oil over medium high heat, pour some of the batter, spread in the pan, cook for 1 minute, flip, cook for 2 minutes more and transfer pancake to a plate.
4. Repeat with the rest of the batter.
5. You will obtain 10 pancakes.
6. Heat up a pan with 1/2 tbsp. coconut oil over medium high heat, add bacon, cook until it's crispy, transfer to paper towels, drain grease and leave it aside in a bowl for now.
7. In another bowl; whisk 8 eggs with some black pepper.
8. Heat up a pan with 1 tbsp. oil over medium high heat, add whisked eggs, cook until they are done and then mix them with cooked bacon.
9. Stir everything well and take off heat. Divide this on your pancakes, roll them and serve for breakfast.

Nutrition Facts Per Serving: Calories: 260; Fat: 7; Fiber: 4; Carbs: 5; Protein: 10

Strawberry And Kiwi Breakfast Smoothie

(**Prep + Cook Time**: 10 minutes | **Servings**: 2)

Ingredients:
- 1½ cups kiwi; chopped
- 1½ cups frozen strawberries; chopped
- 8 mint leaves
- 2 cups crushed ice
- 2 oz. water

Instructions:
1. In your blender, mix kiwi with strawberries and mint and pulse well.
2. Add water and crushed ice and pulse again.

Transfer to glasses and serve right away.

Nutrition Facts Per Serving: Calories: 133; Fat: 1; Carbs: 34; Fiber: 4; Sugar: 9; Protein: 1.3

Yummy Sausage Frittata

(Prep + Cook Time: 40 minutes | **Servings**: 4)

Ingredients:
- 10 eggs
- 2 tbsp. melted ghee
- 1 cup spinach; chopped
- 1/2 lb. sausage; chopped
- 1 cup mushrooms; chopped
- 1 small yellow onion; chopped
- A pinch of sea salt
- Black pepper to the taste

Instructions:
1. Heat up a pan with the ghee over medium high heat, add sausage pieces, stir and brown for a couple of minutes.
2. Add onion, mushroom, spinach, a pinch of salt and black pepper to the taste, stir and cook for a few more minutes.
3. Add whisked eggs, spread evenly and stir gently.
4. Place in the oven at 350 °F and bake for 20 minutes. Leave your Paleo breakfast to cool down before slicing and serving it.

Nutrition Facts Per Serving: Calories: 260; Fat: 8; Fiber: 2; Carbs: 4; Protein: 9

Spinach Frittata

(Prep + Cook Time: 50 minutes | **Servings**: 4)

Ingredients:
- 1/2 lb. sausage; ground
- 2 tbsp. ghee
- 1 cup mushrooms; thinly sliced
- 1 cup spinach leaves; chopped
- 10 eggs; whisked
- 1 small yellow onion; finely chopped
- Black pepper to the taste

Instructions:

1. Heat up a pan with the ghee over medium-high heat, add onion and some black pepper, stir and cook until it browns.
2. Add sausage, stir and also cook until it browns. Add spinach and mushrooms and cook for 4 minutes, stirring from time to time.
3. Take the pan off the heat, add eggs, spread evenly, introduce frittata in the oven at 350 °F and bake for 20 minutes.
4. Take frittata out of the oven, leave it aside for a few minutes to cool down, cut, arrange on plates and serve.

Nutrition Facts Per Serving: Calories: 233; Fat: 13; Carbs: 4; Fiber: 1.2; Sugar: 1; Protein: 21

Sweet Potato Waffles

(**Prep + Cook Time**: 20 minutes | **Servings**: 4)

Ingredients:

- 2 sweet potatoes; peeled and finely grated
- 1/2 tsp. nutmeg; ground
- 2 tbsp. melted coconut oil
- 3 eggs
- 1 tsp. cinnamon powder
- Some apple sauce for serving

Instructions:

1. In a bowl; mix eggs with sweet potatoes, coconut oil, cinnamon and nutmeg and whisk very well.
2. Cook waffles in your waffle iron, arrange them on plates and serve with apple sauce drizzled on top.

Nutrition Facts Per Serving: Calories: 227; Fat: 6; Carbs: 37; Fiber: 2; Sugar: 9; Protein: 6

Paleo Blueberry Muffins

(**Prep + Cook Time**: 35 minutes | **Servings**: 10)

Ingredients:

- 1/2 tsp. baking soda

- 2½ cups almond flour
- 1 tbsp. vanilla extract
- 1/4 cup coconut oil
- 1/4 cup coconut milk
- 2 eggs
- 1/4 cup maple syrup
- 1 tbsp. coconut flour
- 3 tbsp. cinnamon powder
- 1 cup blueberries

Instructions:
1. In a bowl; mix almond flour with baking soda and coconut flour and stir.
2. Add eggs, oil, coconut milk, cinnamon, maple syrup, vanilla and blueberries and stir everything using your mixer.
3. Divide this into muffin cups, place in the oven at 350 °F and bake for 25 minutes. Leave your muffins to cool down a bit, divide between plates and serve them for breakfast.

Nutrition Facts Per Serving: Calories: 240; Fat: 3; Fiber: 1; Carbs: 3; Protein: 1

Eggplant French Toast

(**Prep + Cook Time**: 10 minutes | **Servings**: 2)
Ingredients:
- 1 eggplant; peeled and sliced
- 1 tsp. vanilla extract
- 2 eggs
- Stevia to the taste
- 1 tsp. coconut oil
- A pinch of cinnamon

Instructions:
1. In a bowl; mix eggs with vanilla, stevia and cinnamon and whisk well.
2. Heat up a pan with the coconut oil over medium-high heat.

3. Dip eggplant slices in eggs mix, add to heated pan and cook until they become golden on each side. Arrange them on plates and serve.

Nutrition Facts Per Serving: Calories: 125; Fat: 5; Protein: 7.8; Carbs: 13; Fiber: 7.8

Avocado Muffins

(**Prep + Cook Time**: 40 minutes | **Servings**: 12)
Ingredients:
- 6 thin bacon slices; chopped
- 1 yellow onion; chopped
- 4 avocados; pitted, peeled and chopped
- 4 eggs
- 1/2 cup coconut flour
- 1 cup coconut milk
- 1/2 tsp. baking soda
- A pinch of sea salt
- Black pepper to the taste

Instructions:
1. Heat up a pan over medium high heat, add bacon and onion, stir well and cook until they brown.
2. Meanwhile; put avocado in a bowl and mash with a fork.
3. Add eggs, a pinch of salt, black pepper, milk, baking soda and coconut flour and stir everything well.
4. Add almost all of the bacon and onions, stir well again and divide into muffin pans.
5. Sprinkle the rest of the bacon and onions on top, place in the oven at 350 °F and bake for 20 minutes. Leave your avocado muffins to cool down before dividing them on plates and serving.

Nutrition Facts Per Serving: Calories: 240; Fat: 4; Fiber: 4; Carbs: 7; Protein: 3

Breakfast Burrito

(Prep + Cook Time: 17 minutes | **Servings**: 4)

Ingredients:

- **1 small yellow onion; finely chopped**
- **4 eggs; egg yolks and whites separated**
- **1/4 cup canned green chilies; chopped**
- **2 tomatoes; chopped**
- **1 red bell pepper; cut into thin strips**
- **1/4 cup cilantro; finely chopped**
- **1/2 cup chicken meat; already cooked and shredded**
- **Black pepper to the taste**
- **A drizzle of extra virgin olive oil**
- **1 avocado; pitted, peeled and chopped**
- Hot sauce for serving

Instructions:

1. Put egg whites in a bowl; add some black pepper, whisk them well and leave them aside for now.
2. Heat up a pan with a drizzle of oil over medium-high heat, add half of the egg whites, spread evenly, cook for 30 seconds, cover pan, cook for 1 minute and then slide on a plate.
3. Repeat this with the rest of the egg whites and leave the two "tortillas" aside.
4. Heat up the same pan with another drizzle of oil over medium-high heat, add onions, stir and cook for 1 minute.
5. Add red bell pepper, green chilies, tomato, meat and cilantro and stir.
6. Add egg yolks to the pan and scramble the whole mix.
7. Add avocado, stir; take off heat and spread evenly on the two egg whites "tortillas". Roll them, arrange on plates and serve with some hot sauce.

Nutrition Facts Per Serving: Calories: 170; Fat: 5; Carbs: 1; Sugar: 0.6; Fiber: 0; Protein: 6

Orange And Vanilla Breakfast Delight

(**Prep + Cook Time**: 10 minutes | **Servings**: 2)

Ingredients:

- 2 cups coconut milk
- 1/2 cup chia seeds
- Juice from 1/4 lemon
- Zest from 1 orange
- 1 tbsp. vanilla extract
- 1 tbsp. maple syrup

Instructions:

1. Divide coconut milk, lemon juice, chia, orange zest, vanilla extract and maple syrup into 2 breakfast bowls.
2. Stir well and keep in the fridge until you serve them.

Nutrition Facts Per Serving: Calories: 200; Fat: 3; Fiber: 2; Carbs: 5; Protein: 4

Peach And Coconut Smoothie

(**Prep + Cook Time**: 5 minutes | **Servings**: 2)

Ingredients:

- 1 cup ice
- 2 peaches; peeled and chopped
- Lemon zest to the taste
- 1 cup cold coconut milk
- 1 drop lemon essential oil

Instructions:

1. In your kitchen blender, mix coconut milk with ice and peaches and pulse a few times.
2. Add lemon zest to the taste and 1 drop lemon essential oil and pulse a few more time. Pour into glasses and serve right away.

Nutrition Facts Per Serving: Calories: 200; Fat: 5; Fiber: 4; Carbs: 6; Protein: 8

Easy Spicy Eggs

(**Prep + Cook Time**: 35 minutes | **Servings**: 4)

Ingredients:
- 4 bacon slices; cooked and crumbled
- 12 cherry tomatoes; halved
- 1/2 tsp. turmeric
- 1/2 onion; chopped
- 5 eggs
- 2 Serrano peppers; chopped
- 1 green bell pepper; chopped
- Black pepper to the taste
- A pinch of sea salt

Instructions:
1. In a bowl; whisk eggs with a pinch of salt, black pepper, Serrano peppers, green pepper and turmeric.
2. Heat up a pan over medium heat, add bacon, stir and cook for 3 minutes.
3. Add onion, stir and cook for 2 minutes more.
4. Add eggs and tomatoes, stir; cook for 6 minutes and then bake in the oven at 350 °F for 15 minutes. Leave your eggs to cool down before slicing and serving it.

Nutrition Facts Per Serving: Calories: 240; Fat: 8; Fiber: 3; Carbs: 6; Protein: 8

Paleo Apple Omelet

(**Prep + Cook Time**: 25 minutes | **Servings**: 1)

Ingredients:
- 1 apple; peeled, cored and sliced
- 2 tsp. ghee
- 3 tsp. maple syrup

- 1/2 tsp. cinnamon powder
- 2 eggs; whites and yolks separated
- 2 tbsp. almond milk
- A pinch of sea salt
- Black pepper to the taste
- 2 tbsp. walnuts; toasted and chopped

Instructions:

1. Heat up a pan with half of the ghee over medium high heat, add apple slices and cook them for about 5 minutes.
2. Sprinkle them with cinnamon, drizzle maple syrup, stir gently, cook for 1 minute, transfer them to a plate and leave aside for now.
3. In a bowl; whisk egg yolks with milk, a pinch of salt and black pepper and leave aside for now.
4. In another bowl; whisk egg whites well using your mixer.
5. Combine egg yolks with egg whites.
6. Heat up a pan with the rest of the ghee over medium heat, add eggs mix, stir and cook for 3 minutes.
7. Add apple slices, cover pan, cook eggs for 6 minutes more and transfer everything to a plate. Top with walnuts and serve.

Nutrition Facts Per Serving: Calories: 150; Fat: 1; Fiber: 3; Carbs: 4; Protein: 12

Special Paleo Burrito

(**Prep + Cook Time**: 25 minutes | **Servings**: 2)

Ingredients:

- 1/4 cup canned green chilies; chopped
- 1 small yellow onion; chopped
- 4 eggs; egg yolks and whites divided
- 1/4 cup cilantro; chopped
- 1 red bell pepper; finely cut in strips
- 2 tomatoes; chopped
- 1/2 cup beef; ground and browned for 10 minutes
- 1 avocado; peeled, pitted and chopped

- Some hot sauce for serving
- A drizzle of olive oil

Instructions:
1. Heat up a pan with a drizzle of olive oil over medium high heat, add half of the egg whites after you've whisked them in a bowl; spread evenly and cook for 1 minute.
2. Flip them cook for 1 minute more, transfer to a plate and repeat the action with the rest of the egg whites.
3. Heat up the same pan over medium high heat, add onions, stir and cook for 1 minute.
4. Add chilies, bell pepper, tomato, meat and cilantro, stir and cook for 5 minutes. Add egg yolks, stir well and cook until they are done.
5. Arrange egg whites tortillas on 2 plates, divide eggs and meat mix between them, add some chopped avocado and hot sauce, roll and serve them for breakfast.

Nutrition Facts Per Serving: Calories: 255; Fat: 23; Fiber: 3; Carbs: 7; Protein: 12

Banana Pancakes

(**Prep + Cook Time**: 20 minutes | **Servings**: 2)

Ingredients:
- 2 bananas; peeled and chopped
- 1/4 tsp. baking powder
- 4 eggs
- Cooking spray

Instructions:
1. In a bowl; mix eggs with chopped bananas and baking powder and whisk well.
2. Transfer this to your food processor and blend very well. Heat up a pan over medium high heat after you've sprayed it with some cooking oil.

3. Add some of the pancakes batter, spread in the pan, cook for 1 minute, flip and cook for 30 seconds and transfer to a plate.
4. Repeat this with the rest of the batter, arrange pancakes on plates and serve.

Nutrition Facts Per Serving: 120; Fat: 2; Carbs: 2; Sugar: 1; Protein: 4

Special Breakfast Dish

(**Prep + Cook Time**: 45 minutes | **Servings**: 8)

Ingredients:
- 1 lb. pork meat; ground
- 1 lb. chorizo; ground
- A pinch of sea salt
- Black pepper to the taste
- 8 eggs
- 3 tbsp. ghee
- 1 avocado; pitted, peeled and chopped
- 1 tomato; chopped
- 1/2 cup red onion; chopped
- 2 tbsp. Paleo enchilada sauce

Instructions:
1. In a bowl; mix pork with chorizo, a pinch of salt and black pepper and stir well.
2. Spread this on a lined baking sheet, shape a circle out of it and spread enchilada sauce all over.
3. Place in the oven and be at 350 °F for 25 minutes.
4. Heat up a pan with the ghee over medium heat, add eggs, stir and scramble them.
5. Spread them over pork mix and then add onion, tomato and avocado. Divide between plates and serve.

Nutrition Facts Per Serving: Calories: 345; Fat: 23; Fiber: 3; Carbs: 6; Protein: 23

Breakfast Sandwich

(**Prep + Cook Time**: 20 minutes | **Servings**: 2)

Ingredients:

- 3.5 oz. pumpkin flesh; peeled
- 4 slices paleo coconut bread
- 1 small avocado; pitted and peeled
- 1 carrot; finely grated
- 1 lettuce leaf; torn into 4 pieces

Instructions:

1. Put pumpkin in a tray, introduce in the oven at 350 °F and bake for 10 minutes.
2. Take pumpkin out of the oven, leave aside for 2-3 minutes, transfer to a bowl and mash it a bit. Put avocado in another bowl and also mash it with a fork.
3. Spread avocado on 2 bread slices, add grated carrot, mashed pumpkin and 2 lettuce pieces on each and top them with the rest of the bread slices.

Nutrition Facts Per Serving: Calories: 340; Fat: 7; Protein: 4; Carbs: 13; Fiber: 8; Sugar: 4

Pumpkin Muffins

(**Prep + Cook Time**: 35 minutes | **Servings**: 10)

Ingredients:

- 1¼ cup almond meal
- 2 tbsp. flax meal
- 1 tbsp. flax seeds
- 3/4 cup coconut flour
- 1 tsp. baking soda
- 2 tsp. pumpkin pie spice
- 1/2 tsp. nutmeg; ground
- 1/2 tsp. ginger powder
- 5 eggs
- 1/4 cup coconut oil
- 1/4 cup agave

- 1 cup pumpkin puree
- 1 cup blueberries
- 1 cup walnuts; chopped

Instructions:

1. In a bowl; mix almond meal with flax meal, flax seeds, coconut flour, baking soda, nutmeg, ginger and pumpkin spice and stir.
2. In another bowl; mix eggs with oil, agave, pumpkin puree, walnuts and blueberries and whisk well.
3. Combine the 2 mixtures and stir using your mixer.
4. Divide this into a lined muffin tray, place in the oven at 350 °F and bake for 25 minutes. Leave your muffins to cool down, divide them between plates and serve.

Nutrition Facts Per Serving: Calories: 240; Fat: 3; Fiber: 2; Carbs: 4; Protein: 6

Portobello Sandwich

(**Prep + Cook Time**: 15 minutes | **Servings**: 1)

Ingredients:

- 2 Portobello mushroom caps
- Some lettuce leaves
- 2 avocado slices
- 1/2 lb. bacon; chopped

Instructions:

1. Heat up a pan over medium high heat, add bacon, cook until it's crispy, transfer to paper towels and drain grease.
2. Heat up the pan with the bacon fat over medium high heat, add mushroom caps, cook for 2 minutes on each side and take off heat.
3. Put 1 mushroom cap on a plate, add bacon, avocado slices and lettuce leaves, top with the other mushroom cap and serve.

Nutrition Facts Per Serving: Calories: 200; Fat: 4; Fiber: 2; Carbs: 4; Protein: 6

Spinach Omelet

Ingredients:

- 2 eggs; whisked
- 1 tbsp. ghee; melted
- A pinch of black pepper
- 1 handful baby spinach; torn
- 1 onion; chopped
- 4 thyme springs; chopped
- 3 garlic cloves; minced
- 1 red bell pepper; chopped
- 1 green bell pepper; chopped
- 3 tbsp. olive oil
- 1 cup cherry tomatoes; halved
- 1 red chili pepper; chopped

Instructions:

1. Heat up a pan with the ghee over medium high heat, add eggs, black pepper, stir a bit, cook until eggs are done, add spinach, stir gently, cook for a few minutes and divide between plates.
2. Heat up another pan with the oil over medium high heat, add onion, stir and cook for 3 minutes.
3. Add garlic, stir and cook for 1 minute more. Add thyme, tomatoes, red, yellow pepper and chili pepper, stir; cook for 5 minutes more and divide on top of the omelet. Serve hot.

Nutrition Facts Per Serving: Calories: 200; Fat: 5; Fiber: 3; Carbs: 4; Protein: 4

Breakfast Sliders

(**Prep + Cook Time**: 25 minutes | **Servings**: 3)

Ingredients:

- 3 Portobello mushroom caps
- 4 bacon slices

- 3 eggs
- 4 oz. smoked salmon

Instructions:

1. Heat up a pan over medium high heat, add bacon, cook until it's crispy, transfer to paper towels and drain grease.
2. Heat up the pan with the bacon grease over medium heat and place egg rings in it.
3. Crack and egg in each, cook them for 6 minutes and transfer them to a plate.
4. Heat up the pan again over medium high heat, add mushroom caps, cook the for 5 minutes and transfer them to a platter. Top each mushroom cap with bacon, salmon and eggs. Serve hot.

Nutrition Facts Per Serving: Calories: 180; Fat: 3; Fiber: 5; Carbs: 7; Protein: 8

Delicious Wrapped Eggs

(**Prep + Cook Time**: 25 minutes | **Servings**: 2)

Ingredients:

- 4 bacon slices
- 2 bacon slices; chopped
- 4 eggs
- 1/2 yellow onion; chopped
- 1 sweet potato; peeled and chopped
- 1 tbsp. olive oil
- A pinch of sea salt
- Black pepper to the taste

Instructions:

1. Heat up a pan over medium high heat, add 4 bacon slices , cook until it's crispy, transfer to paper towels, drain grease and line 4 muffin molds with it.
2. Crack an egg into each bacon cup, season with salt and pepper, place in the oven at 375 °F and bake for 15 minutes.

3. Meanwhile; heat up a pan with the oil over medium high heat, add onion and sweet potato, stir and cook for a few minutes.
4. Add the rest of the bacon, stir and cook for a few more minutes. Divide wrapped eggs on plates, add sweet potato mix on the side and serve.

Nutrition Facts Per Serving: Calories: 200; Fat: 5; Fiber: 3; Carbs: 6; Protein: 5

Coconut Pancakes

(Prep + Cook Time: 20 minutes | **Servings**: 8)

Ingredients:
- 1/4 cup coconut milk
- 1/4 cup coconut flour
- 1/8 tsp. baking soda
- 3 eggs
- 2 tbsp. coconut oil
- 1/2 tsp. vanilla extract
- 2 tbsp. honey
- Maple syrup for serving
- 2 tbsp. melted ghee

Instructions:
1. In a bowl; whisk eggs with honey and coconut oil. Add vanilla, coconut milk, baking soda and coconut flour and stir very well.
2. Heat up a pan with the ghee over medium heat, add some of the batter, spread into the pan, cook until it's golden, flip and cook on the other side as well.
3. Repeat with the rest of the batter, divide your pancakes between plates and serve with maple syrup on top.

Nutrition Facts Per Serving: Calories: 300; Fat: 5; Fiber: 2; Carbs: 4; Protein: 10

Paleo Kale Frittata

(**Prep + Cook Time**: 40 minutes | **Servings**: 4)

Ingredients:

- 3 bacon slices; cooked and crumbled
- 1/3 cup yellow onion; chopped
- 1 tbsp. coconut oil
- 1/2 cup red bell pepper; chopped
- 2 cups kale; torn
- 1/2 cup almond milk
- 8 eggs
- A pinch of black pepper

Instructions:

1. In a bowl; whisk eggs with some black pepper and almond milk.
2. Heat up a pan with the oil over medium high heat, add bell pepper and onion, stir and cook for 3 minutes.
3. Add kale, stir; cover pan and cook for 5 minutes more.
4. Uncover your pan, add bacon and eggs, spread evenly around the pan and cook for 4 minutes.
5. Introduce your pan in the oven at 350 °F and bake for 15 minutes. Take frittata out of the oven, leave it to cool down a bit before cutting and serving it for breakfast.

Nutrition Facts Per Serving: Calories: 240; Fat: 13; Fiber: 2; Carbs: 5; Protein: 15

Ham And Mushroom Paleo Breakfast

(**Prep + Cook Time**: 20 minutes | **Servings**: 1)

Ingredients:

- 2 tbsp. ghee
- 1/4 cup coconut milk
- 3 eggs
- 3.5 oz. smoked ham; chopped
- 3 oz. mushrooms; sliced

- 1 cup arugula; torn
- A pinch of black pepper

Instructions:
1. Heat up a pan with half of the ghee over medium heat, add mushrooms, stir and cook for 3 minutes.
2. Add ham, stir; cook for 2-3 minutes more and transfer everything to a plate.
3. In a bowl; mix eggs with coconut milk and black pepper and whisk well.
4. Heat up the pan with the rest of the ghee over medium heat, add eggs, spread into the pan, cook for a couple of minutes, start stirring and cook until eggs are completely done.
5. Transfer this to a serving bowl; add mushrooms mix on top and arugula. Toss everything to coat well and serve right away.

Nutrition Facts Per Serving: Calories: 356; Fat: 23; Fiber: 2; Carbs: 6; Protein: 25

Tasty Bacon Muffins

(**Prep + Cook Time:** 40 minutes | **Servings:** 4)

Ingredients:
- 4 oz. bacon slices
- 3 garlic cloves; minced
- 1 small yellow onion; chopped
- 1 zucchini; thinly sliced
- A handful spinach; torn
- 6 canned and pickled artichoke hearts; chopped
- 8 eggs
- 1/4 tsp. paprika
- A pinch of black pepper
- A pinch of cayenne pepper
- 1/4 cup coconut cream

Instructions:

1. Heat up a pan over medium high heat, add bacon, stir; cook until it's crispy, transfer to paper towels, drain grease and leave aside for now.
2. Heat up the same pan over medium heat again, add garlic and onion, stir and cook for 4 minutes.
3. In a bowl; mix eggs with coconut cream, onions, garlic, paprika, black pepper and cayenne and whisk well.
4. Add spinach, zucchini and artichoke pieces and stir everything.
5. Divide crispy bacon slices in a muffin pan, add eggs mixture on top, introduce your muffins in the oven and bake at 400 °F for 20 minutes. Leave them to cool down before serving them for breakfast.

Nutrition Facts Per Serving: Calories: 270; Fat: 12; Fiber: 4; Carbs: 6; Protein: 12

Simple Paleo Burger

(**Prep + Cook Time**: 30 minutes | **Servings**: 4)

Ingredients:
- 8 bacon slices; chopped and cooked
- 5 eggs
- 1 lb. beef; ground
- 1/2 cup sausage; ground
- 3 sun-dried tomatoes; chopped
- 2 tbsp. almond meal
- 2 tsp. basil
- 2 tbsp. coconut oil
- 1 tsp. garlic; minced

Instructions:
1. In a bowl; mix beef with garlic, basil, tomatoes, almond meal and 1 egg, stir well and shape 4 burgers.
2. Heat up a grill over medium high heat, add burgers, cook them for 5 minutes on each side, transfer to plates and leave them aside.

3. Heat up a pan over medium high heat, add sausage, cook until it's done and divide into burgers. Add cooked bacon on top of sausages and leave aside for now.
4. Heat up a pan with the coconut oil over medium high heat, crack one egg at a time, fry them well and divide them on burgers.

Nutrition Facts Per Serving: Calories: 340; Fat: 20; Fiber: 3; Carbs: 7; Protein: 20

Tasty Chicken Waffles

(Prep + Cook Time: 20 minutes | **Servings**: 4)
Ingredients:
- 1½ cups chicken; cooked and shredded
- 1/2 cup hot sauce
- 1 cup almond flour
- 2 green onions; chopped
- 1/2 cup tapioca flour
- 2 eggs
- 6 tbsp. coconut flour
- A pinch of cayenne pepper
- 3/4 tsp. baking soda
- 1 tsp. garlic powder
- 1 cup coconut milk
- 1/4 cup ghee+ some more for the waffle iron
- A pinch of sea salt

Instructions:
1. In a bowl; mix almond flour with tapioca flour, coconut one, baking soda, garlic powder and a pinch of salt and stir well.
2. Add chicken, hot sauce, green onions, eggs, milk and 1/4 cup ghee and blend using your mixer.
3. Pour some of the batter into your greased waffle iron, close the lid and make your waffle. Repeat with the rest of the batter, divide waffles between plates and serve them in the morning.

Nutrition Facts Per Serving: Calories: 200; Fat: 11; Fiber: 1; Carbs: 7; Protein: 8

Zucchini And Chocolate Muffins

(**Prep + Cook Time**: 40 minutes | **Servings**: 8)

Ingredients:

- 4 eggs
- 1/4 cup honey
- 1/4 cup melted ghee
- 1/4 cup coconut milk
- 1/4 cup coconut flour
- 1/2 cup almond flour
- 1 tsp. baking soda
- 1/4 cup cocoa powder
- 1 zucchini; grated
- 4 oz. dark chocolate; chopped
- 1 tsp. vanilla extract

Instructions:

1. In a bowl; mix eggs with ghee and whisk using a mixer.
2. Add coconut milk, honey and vanilla and whisk well again.
3. In another bowl; mix coconut flour with baking soda, almond flour and cocoa powder and stir well.
4. Combine the 2 mixtures and stir again.
5. Add chocolate pieces and zucchini, stir gently, divide into a lined muffin tray and bake in the oven at 350 °F for 30 minutes. Serve your muffins cold.

Nutrition Facts Per Serving: Calories: 230; Fat: 4; Fiber: 2; Carbs: 4; Protein: 6

Beef And Squash Skillet

(**Prep + Cook Time**: 30 minutes | **Servings**: 3)

Ingredients:

- 15 oz. beef; ground

- 2 tbsp. ghee
- 3 garlic cloves; minced
- 2 celery stalks; chopped
- 1 yellow onion; chopped
- A pinch of sea salt
- White pepper to the taste
- 1/2 tsp. coriander; ground
- 1 tsp. cumin; ground
- 1 tsp. garam masala
- 1/2 butternut squash; chopped and already cooked
- 3 eggs
- 1 small avocado; peeled, pitted and chopped
- 15 oz. spinach

Instructions:
1. Put spinach in a heatproof bowl; place in your microwave and cook for 1 minute.
2. Squeeze spinach and leave it aside.
3. Heat up a pan with the ghee over medium heat, add onion, garlic, celery, a pinch of salt and white pepper, stir and cook for 3 minutes.
4. Add beef, cumin, garam masala and coriander, stir and cook for a few minutes more.
5. Add squash flesh and spinach, stir and make 3 holes in this mix.
6. Crack an egg into each, cover pan, place in the oven at 375 °F and bake for 15 minutes. Divide this mix on plates and serve with avocado on top.

Nutrition Facts Per Serving: Calories: 400; Fat: 23; Fiber: 7; Carbs: 8; Protein: 24

Chorizo Paleo Breakfast Skillet

(**Prep + Cook Time**: 40 minutes | **Servings**: 2)
Ingredients:
- **1 small avocado; peeled, pitted and chopped**

- **1/2 cup beef stock**
- **1 lb. chorizo; chopped**
- **2 poblano peppers; chopped**
- **1 cup kale; chopped**
- **8 mushrooms; chopped**
- **1/2 yellow onion; chopped**
- **3 garlic cloves; minced**
- **1/2 cup cilantro; chopped**
- **4 bacon slices; chopped**
- 4 eggs

Instructions:

1. Heat up a pan over medium heat, add chorizo and bacon, stir and cook until they are browned.
2. Add garlic, peppers and onions, stir and cook for 6 minutes more.
3. Add stock, mushrooms and kale, stir and cook for 4 minutes more.
4. Make holes in this mix, crack an egg in each, place in the oven at 350 °F and bake for 12 minutes. Divide this mix on plates, sprinkle cilantro and avocado on top and serve.

Nutrition Facts Per Serving: Calories: 200; Fat: 6; Fiber: 3; Carbs: 6; Protein: 10

Delicious Bacon Waffles

(**Prep + Cook Time**: 40 minutes | **Servings**: 4)

Ingredients:

- 2 eggs
- 6 bacon slices
- 1/2 cup coconut milk
- 1 tsp. vanilla extract
- 2 tbsp. maple syrup
- 1/2 tsp. baking soda
- 1¾ cups almond flour

- 2 tbsp. ghee
- Maple syrup for serving

Instructions:
1. Place bacon slices on a lined baking sheet, place in the oven at 400 °F and bake for 20 minutes.
2. Transfer bacon to paper towels, drain grease, crumble them and leave them aside.
3. In a bowl; mix almond flour with baking soda.
4. In another bowl; whisk eggs with vanilla extract, ghee, 2 tbsp. maple syrup and coconut milk.
5. Combine the wet and dry mixtures and stir well.
6. Add crumbled bacon, stir again and pour some of the batter in your waffle iron.
7. Close the lid, cook your waffle for 5 minutes and transfer it to a plate. Repeat with the rest of the batter, divide waffles between plates and serve them with maple syrup on top.

Nutrition Facts Per Serving: Calories: 200; Fat: 12; Fiber: 4; Carbs: 7; Protein: 10

Paleo Porridge

(**Prep + Cook Time**: 16 minutes | **Servings**: 3)

Ingredients:
- 1 big plantain; peeled and mashed
- 1/4 cup flax meal
- 2 cups coconut milk
- 3/4 cup almond meal
- 1 tsp. cinnamon; powder
- A pinch of cloves; ground
- 1/2 tsp. ginger powder
- A pinch of nutmeg; ground
- Maple syrup for serving
- Some unsweetened coconut flakes for serving

Instructions:

1. In a small pan, mix plantain with flax meal, almond meal, coconut milk, cinnamon, cloves, ginger and nutmeg, stir well, bring to a simmer over medium heat and cook for about 6 minutes.
2. Divide your porridge into bowls, top with coconut flakes and maple syrup and serve.

Nutrition Facts Per Serving: Calories: 140; Fat: 3; Fiber: 2; Carbs: 5; Protein: 6

Delicious Steak And Veggie Paleo Breakfast

(**Prep + Cook Time**: 35 minutes | **Servings**: 4)

Ingredients:
- 2 sweet potatoes; chopped
- 3/4 lb. sirloin steak; cut into small pieces
- 1 yellow onion; chopped
- 1 green bell pepper; chopped
- 1 red bell pepper; chopped
- 2 tbsp. bacon fat
- Black pepper to the taste
- A pinch of sea salt
- 1 tomato; sliced
- 4 eggs

Instructions:
1. Heat up a pan with half of the fat over medium high heat, add steak, cook for a few minutes until it browns and takes off heat.
2. Heat up the same pan with the rest of the fat over medium high heat, add green and red peppers and onions, stir and cook for 5 minutes. Add sweet potatoes, stir and cook for 10 minutes more.
3. Add steak pieces, stir well, make 4 holes, crack an egg in each, arrange tomato slices, sprinkle black pepper and a pinch of salt, place in the oven at 350 °F and bake for 12 minutes. Serve warm.

Nutrition Facts Per Serving: Calories: 180; Fat: 4; Fiber: 3; Carbs: 6; Protein: 8

Veggie Omelet Cupcakes

(**Prep + Cook Time**: 30 minutes | **Servings**: 4)

Ingredients:
- 4 bacon slices; chopped
- A handful spinach; chopped
- 1 white onion; chopped
- 1 red bell pepper; chopped
- 1 green bell pepper; chopped
- 1 yellow bell pepper; chopped
- 1 tomato; chopped
- 8 eggs
- A pinch of sea salt
- Black pepper to the taste

Instructions:
1. Heat up a pan over medium high heat, add bacon, stir; cook until it's crispy, transfer to paper towels, drain grease and leave aside for now.
2. Heat up the same pan with the bacon fat over medium high heat, add onion, stir and cook for 3 minutes.
3. Add tomato, all bell peppers, a pinch of salt and black pepper, stir; cook for a couple more minutes and take off heat.
4. In a bowl; whisk eggs with a pinch of salt and black pepper and mix with veggies and bacon.
5. Stir, divide this into a lined muffin tray, place in the oven at 350 °F and bake for 17 minutes. Leave you special muffins to cool down, divide between plates and serve.

Nutrition Facts Per Serving: Calories: 200; Fat: 4; Fiber: 2; Carbs: 5; Protein: 7

Apple Pancakes

(**Prep + Cook Time**: 30 minutes | **Servings**: 18)

Ingredients:
- 2 cups apples; peeled, cored and chopped
- 1 tbsp. coconut oil
- 4 eggs
- 2 tsp. cinnamon powder
- 2 tbsp. honey
- 1 cup almond milk+ 3 tablespoons
- 1 tsp. vanilla extract
- 1/2 cup coconut flour
- A pinch of nutmeg
- 1/2 tsp. baking soda
- 3 tbsp. ghee
- 2 tbsp. maple syrup

Instructions:
1. Heat up a pan with 1 tbsp. oil over medium heat, add apples and cinnamon, stir and cook for 5 minutes.
2. In a bowl; whisk eggs with vanilla, 1 cup milk, honey, baking soda, coconut flour and nutmeg and whisk. Add apples and the rest of the almond milk and stir again well.
3. Heat up a pan with the ghee over medium high heat, pour some of the pancake batter, spread, cook until it's done on one side, flip, cook on the other side as well and transfer to a plate.
4. Repeat with the rest of the batter and serve your pancakes with maple syrup on top.

Nutrition Facts Per Serving: Calories: 340; Fat: 14; Fiber: 4; Carbs: 7; Protein: 12

Bacon And Egg Breakfast Sandwich

(**Prep + Cook Time**: 20 minutes | **Servings**: 2)
Ingredients:
- 2 cups bell peppers; chopped
- 1/2 tbsp. avocado oil
- 3 eggs

- 4 bacon slices

Instructions:
1. Heat up a pan with the oil over medium high heat, add bell peppers, stir and cook until they are soft.
2. Heat up another pan over medium heat, add bacon, stir and cook until it's crispy.
3. In a bowl; whisk eggs really well and add them to bell peppers.
4. Cook until eggs are done for about 8 minutes. Divide half of the bacon slices between plates, add eggs, top with bacon slices and serve.

Nutrition Facts Per Serving: Calories: 200; Fat: 4; Fiber: 3; Carbs: 6; Protein: 10

Side Dish Recipes

Roasted Bell Peppers

(**Prep + Cook Time**: 1 hour 10 minutes | **Servings**: 4)

Ingredients:
- 6 bell peppers (green; yellow and red)
- 1 garlic clove; finely minced
- 2 tbsp. capers
- 2 tbsp. extra virgin olive oil
- 1/4 cup red wine vinegar
- A pinch of sea salt
- Black pepper to the taste
- 2 tbsp. parsley; finely chopped

Instructions:
1. Arrange bell peppers on a lined baking sheet, introduce them in the oven at 400 °F and bake for 40 minutes.
2. Transfer bell peppers to a bowl; cover and leave them aside for 15 minutes.

3. Peel bell peppers, discard seeds, cut into strips and transfer them to a bowl.
4. Add a pinch of sea salt and pepper to the taste, vinegar, oil, garlic, capers and parsley and toss to coat. Divide between plates and serve as a side dish.

Nutrition Facts Per Serving: Calories: 98; Fat: 1; Carbs: 10; Fiber: 3; Sugar: 2; Protein: 2

Paleo Ginger Cauliflower Rice

(**Prep + Cook Time**: 20 minutes | **Servings**: 4)

Ingredients:
- 5 cups cauliflower florets
- 3 tbsp. coconut oil
- 4 ginger slices; grated
- 1 tbsp. coconut vinegar
- 3 garlic cloves; minced
- 1 tbsp. chives; minced
- A pinch of sea salt
- Black pepper to the taste

Instructions:
1. Put cauliflower florets in a food processor and pulse well.
2. Heat up a pan with the oil over medium high heat, add ginger, stir and cook for 3 minutes.
3. Add cauliflower and garlic, stir and cook for 7 minutes. Add a pinch of salt, black pepper, vinegar and chives, stir; cook for a few seconds more, divide between plates and serve.

Nutrition Facts Per Serving: Calories: 100; Fat: 2; Fiber: 5; Carbs: 6; Protein: 8

Roasted Beets

(**Prep + Cook Time**: 1 hour 10 minutes | **Servings**: 4)

Ingredients:
- 2 tbsp. extra virgin olive oil
- 6 beets; cut into quarters and then thinly sliced
- A pinch of sea salt

- Black pepper to the taste
- 1/2 cup balsamic vinegar
- 1 tsp. orange zest
- 2 tsp. maple syrup

Instructions:

1. Arrange beets on a lined baking sheet, add a pinch of salt and pepper and the olive oil, toss to coat well, introduce in preheated oven at 325 °F and roast for 45 minutes.
2. Heat up a pan over medium heat, add vinegar and maple syrup, stir well, cook until vinegar is reduced and take off heat.
3. Take beets out of the oven, leave them to cool down a bit, transfer to plates, drizzle the glaze on top, sprinkle orange zest and serve right away as a side dish.

Nutrition Facts Per Serving: Calories: 80; Fat: 1; Carbs: 8; Fiber: 2; Sugar: 7; Protein: 2

Asparagus Side Dish

(**Prep + Cook Time**: 20 minutes | **Servings**: 4)

Ingredients:

- 1/4 cup caramelized pecans; chopped
- 4 bacon slices; already cooked and crumbled
- 1½ lbs. asparagus
- A pinch of sea salt
- Black pepper to the taste
- 2 garlic cloves; minced
- 1 shallot; finely chopped
- 1/2 tsp. red chili flakes
- 2 tsp. mustard
- 1 tsp. maple syrup
- 2 tbsp. ghee
- 2 tsp. balsamic vinegar

Instructions:

1. In a bowl; mix vinegar with mustard, maple syrup, sea salt and pepper to the taste and stir well.
2. Heat up a pan with the ghee over medium high heat, add garlic, shallots and pepper flakes, stir and cook for 2 minutes.
3. Add asparagus, stir and cook for 5 minutes.
4. Add vinegar mix and more pepper, toss to coat and cook for 3 minutes more. Transfer to plates, top with bacon and pecans and serve as a side dish.

Nutrition Facts Per Serving: Calories: 80; Fat: 4; Carbs: 4; Fiber: 2; Sugar: 0; Protein: 2

Roasted Cherry Tomatoes

(**Prep + Cook Time**: 25 minutes | **Servings**: 4)
Ingredients:
- 2 tbsp. extra virgin olive oil
- 20 oz. colored cherry tomatoes; cut in halves
- 6 garlic cloves; finely minced
- A pinch of sea salt
- Black pepper to the taste
- 1 tbsp. basil leaves; finely chopped

Instructions:
1. In a large bowl; mix tomatoes with a pinch of sea salt, pepper to the taste, olive oil, garlic and basil and toss to coat.
2. Spread these on a lined baking dish, introduce in the oven at 375 °F and bake for 20 minutes.
3. Take tomatoes out of the oven, leave them to cool down, divide to plates and serve as a side dish for a frittata for example.

Nutrition Facts Per Serving: Calories: 35; Fat: 2.4; Carbs: 2; Fiber: 0.4; Sugar: 0; Protein: 0.4

Roasted Okra

(**Prep + Cook Time**: 35 minutes | **Servings**: 3)

Ingredients:

- 18 okra pods; sliced
- A pinch of sea salt
- Black pepper to the taste
- Sweet paprika to the taste
- 1 tbsp. extra virgin olive oil

Instructions:

1. Put okra in a baking dish, season with, paprika, a pinch of salt and pepper to the taste and drizzle olive oil.
2. Introduce in preheated oven at 425 °F and bake for 15 minutes. Take okra out of the oven, leave them to cool down, divide between plates and serve as a side dish.

Nutrition Facts Per Serving: Calories: 76; Fat: 0.8; Carbs: 16; Fiber: 7.3; Sugar: 2.7; Protein: 4.6

Sweet Potatoes Dish

(**Prep + Cook Time**: 55 minutes | **Servings**: 4)

Ingredients:

- 3 sweet potatoes; pricked with a fork and ends cut off
- A pinch of sea salt
- 1/2 cup coconut milk
- 1/4 cup coconut; toasted and shredded
- 2 tbsp. cilantro; chopped
- Seeds from 1 pomegranate
- 1 lime; cut into wedges

Instructions:

1. Arrange potatoes on a lined baking sheet, introduce in the oven at 400 °F and bake for 45 minutes.
2. Take sweet potatoes out of the oven, leave them to cool down, peel and mash them with a fork and put in a bowl.
3. Add a pinch of sea salt, shredded coconut, coconut milk and pomegranate seeds and stir well. Transfer to plates and serve as a side dish.

Calories: 160; Fat: 1; Carbs: 20; Fiber: 4; Sugar: 2; Protein: 5

Paleo Asparagus And Mushrooms Side Dish

(**Prep + Cook Time**: 20 minutes | **Servings**: 4)

Ingredients:

- 1 lb. asparagus; trimmed
- A pinch of sea salt
- Black pepper to the taste
- 8 green onions; thinly sliced
- 2 tbsp. coconut oil
- 2 tbsp. red wine vinegar
- 2 tbsp. hazelnuts; toasted and chopped
- 1 lb. mushrooms; chopped

Instructions:

1. In a bowl; mix vinegar with a pinch of sea salt, pepper to the taste and half of the oil and whisk well.
2. Put some water in a pot, bring to a boil over medium heat, add asparagus, cook for 3 minutes, drain and transfer to a bowl filled with cold water.
3. Heat up a pan with the rest of the oil over medium-high heat, add mushrooms and cook them for 4-5 minutes stirring from time to time.
4. Add onions, stir and cook for 1 minute.
5. Add drained asparagus, stir; cook 3 more minutes and take off heat.
6. Add vinegar mix, stir and transfer to plates. Sprinkle hazelnuts at the end and serve as a side dish!

Nutrition Facts Per Serving: Calories: 70; Fat: 2.5; Carbs: 7; Fiber: 3.2; Sugar: 2; Protein: 5

French Fries

(**Prep + Cook Time**: 40 minutes | **Servings**: 3)

Ingredients:
- 2 lbs. sweet potatoes; cut into wedges
- A pinch of sea salt
- Black pepper to the taste
- 1/4 cup ghee
- 3 tsp. thyme and rosemary; dried

Instructions:
1. In a bowl; mix potato wedges with ghee, a pinch of salt and pepper to the taste and dried herbs and toss to coat.
2. Spread potatoes on a lined baking sheet and bake in the oven at 425 °F for 25 minutes. Take potatoes out of the oven, leave them aside for 5 minutes, divide between plates and serve as a side dish.

Nutrition Facts Per Serving: Calories: 120; Carbs: 12; Fiber: 4; Sugar: 1; Protein: 12

Roasted Beets

(**Prep + Cook Time**: 1 hour 10 minutes | **Servings**: 4)

Ingredients:
- 2 tbsp. balsamic vinegar
- 8 beets; cut in quarters
- 1 tbsp. melted coconut oil
- 1/4 tsp. truffle salt

Instructions:
1. In a bowl; mix beets with vinegar, oil and truffle salt, toss to coat well and spread them on a lined baking sheet.
2. Introduce beets in the oven at 350 °F and roast them for 1 hour. Divide beets between plates and serve them.

Nutrition Facts Per Serving: Calories: 150; Fat: 3; Fiber: 3; Carbs: 5; Protein: 10

Sautéed Spinach Dish

(**Prep + Cook Time**: 43 minutes | **Servings**: 3)

Ingredients:

- 3 cups spinach; torn
- 3 yellow onions; sliced
- 3 garlic cloves; finely minced
- A pinch of sea salt
- Black pepper to the taste
- 10 mushrooms; sliced
- 1 tbsp. coconut oil
- 1 tbsp. balsamic vinegar
- 1 tbsp. ghee

Instructions:

1. Heat up a pan with the oil and ghee over medium-high heat, add garlic and onions, stir and cook for 10 minutes.
2. Reduce temperature to low and cook onions for 20 minutes, stirring from time to time.
3. Add vinegar, mushrooms, salt and pepper, stir and cook for 10 minutes. Add spinach, stir; cook for 3 minutes more, take off heat, divide among plates and serve.

Nutrition Facts Per Serving: Calories: 89; Fat: 7; Carbs: 3.7; Fiber: 1.4; Sugar: 0.3; Protein: 2

Yummy Kale Dish

(**Prep + Cook Time**: 18 minutes | **Servings**: 4)

Ingredients:

- 3 oz. bacon; chopped
- 1 bunch kale; roughly chopped
- 1/2 cup veggie stock
- 1 tbsp. lemon juice
- 1 garlic clove; minced
- Black pepper to the taste

Instructions:

1. Put bacon in a pan and heat it up over medium high heat.
2. Cook for 3 minutes, stirring all the time.

3. Add kale, stock and black pepper to the taste, stir and cook for 4 minutes. Add lemon juice and garlic, stir; cook for 1 minute more, divide between plates and serve as a side dish.

Nutrition Facts Per Serving: Calories: 150; Fat: 5; Fiber: 2; Carbs: 4; Protein: 3

Slow Cooked Mushrooms

(**Prep + Cook Time**: 4 hours 10 minutes | **Servings**: 4)

Ingredients:
- 4 garlic cloves; finely minced
- 1/4 tsp. thyme; dried
- 1/2 tsp. basil; dried
- 1/2 tsp. oregano; dried
- 24 oz. cremini mushrooms
- 1 bay leaf
- 2 tbsp. parsley leaves; chopped
- 1/4 cup coconut milk
- 1 cup veggie stock
- 2 tbsp. ghee
- Black pepper to the taste
- A pinch of sea salt

Instructions:
1. In your slow cooker, mix mushrooms with garlic, basil, oregano, thyme, parsley and bay leaf.
2. Add coconut milk, ghee, veggie stock, salt and pepper, stir; cover pot and cook on Low for 4 hours.
3. Uncover pot, discard bay leaf, transfer to plates and serve as a side dish.

Nutrition Facts Per Serving: Calories: 100; Fat: 10; Carbs: 6; Sugar: 1; Fiber: 1; Protein: 5

Zucchini And Leeks Side Dish

(**Prep + Cook Time**: 20 minutes | **Servings**: 4)

Ingredients:

- 2 zucchinis, sliced
- 2 leeks, sliced lengthwise
- 1/4 cup extra virgin olive oil
- 1/3 cup walnuts, toasted and chopped
- 1/4 cup cilantro, chopped
- 1/4 cup parsley, chopped
- A pinch of sea salt
- Black pepper to the taste
- Juice of 1 lemon
- 2 garlic cloves, minced

Instructions:
1. Season leeks and zucchinis with a pinch of sea salt and pepper to the taste, arrange them on heated grill over medium-high heat and cook them for 8 minutes, flipping them from time to time.
2. Transfer veggies to a bowl; add walnuts, parsley, oil, cilantro, garlic and lemon. Toss to coat and serve as a side dish.

Nutrition Facts Per Serving: Calories: 120; Fat: 20; Carbs: 12; Sugar: 0; Fiber: 1; Protein: 4

Mashed Cauliflower Dish

(**Prep + Cook Time**: 35 minutes | **Servings**: 4)

Ingredients:
- 4 bacon slices; already cooked and crumbled
- 2 garlic cloves; finely chopped
- 6 cups cauliflower florets
- 2 green onions; thinly sliced
- A pinch of sea salt
- Black pepper to the taste
- 3 tbsp. ghee

Instructions:
1. Put water in a pot, place on stove over medium-high heat and bring to a boil.

109

2. Add cauliflower, cook for 20 minutes, drain water and leave cauliflower in the pot.
3. Add a pinch of salt, pepper to the taste and the ghee and mash everything using a hand mixer. Transfer to plates, sprinkle crumbled bacon and chopped green onions on top and serve as a side dish.

Nutrition Facts Per Serving: Calories: 70; Fat: 15; Carbs: 9; Sugar: 2; Fiber: 3; Protein: 7

Roasted Cabbage Side Dish

(Prep + Cook Time: 40 minutes | **Servings**: 4)

Ingredients:
- 1 green cabbage head; cut into medium wedges
- A pinch of sea salt
- Black pepper to the taste
- A pinch of red chili flakes
- A pinch of garlic powder
- 2 tbsp. extra virgin olive oil
- Juice from 2 lemons

Instructions:
1. Brush cabbage wedges with olive oil, season with a pinch of sea salt and pepper to the taste, sprinkle garlic powder and pepper flakes and arrange them on a lined baking sheet.
2. Introduce in preheated oven at 450 °F and bake for 15 minutes.
3. Flip cabbage wedges, bake for 15 more minutes, take out of the oven and divide them between plates. Serve as a side dish with lemon juice squeezed on top.

Nutrition Facts Per Serving: Calories: 67; Fat: 6; Carbs: 1; Fiber: 2; Protein: 0; Sugar: 0

Roasted Carrots

(Prep + Cook Time: 40 minutes | **Servings**: 4)

Ingredients:
- 1½ lbs. young carrots (yellow; purple and red ones)
- 2 tbsp. balsamic vinegar
- 2 garlic cloves; finely minced
- 2 tbsp. coconut oil; melted
- A pinch of sea salt
- 1 tbsp. honey
- Black pepper to the taste
- A handful parsley leaves; finely chopped

Instructions:
1. In a bowl; mix vinegar with oil, honey, garlic, a pinch of salt and pepper to the taste and stir very well.
2. Add carrots and toss to coat. Transfer this to a baking dish, introduce in the oven at 400 °F and bake for 30 minutes.
3. Take carrots out of the oven, sprinkle parsley on top, toss gently and serve right away as a side dish.

Nutrition Facts Per Serving: Calories: 40; Carbs: 20; Protein: 2; Fat: 6; Sugar: 1; Fiber: 1

Pumpkin Fries

(**Prep + Cook Time**: 45 minutes | **Servings**: 4)

Ingredients:
- 1 big pumpkin; peeled and cut in medium fries
- 1 tbsp. sriracha sauce
- 1 tbsp. maple syrup
- 1 tbsp. coconut oil; melted

Instructions:
1. Drizzle the oil on a lined baking sheet, add pumpkin fries and toss them well.
2. Add maple syrup and sriracha, toss to coat well again, place in the oven at 400 °F and bake for 35 minutes.
3. Divide pumpkin fries between plates and serve them as a Paleo side dish.

Nutrition Facts Per Serving: Calories: 60; Fat: 2; Fiber: 1; Carbs: 1; Protein: 1

Paleo Veggie Mix

(Prep + Cook Time: 1 hour 40 minutes | **Servings**: 8)

Ingredients:
- 1 lb. yellow squash; peeled and chopped
- 1 yellow onion; chopped
- 3 tbsp. olive oil
- 2 garlic cloves; minced
- 2 cups chicken stock
- 4 lbs. mixed sweet potatoes; parsnips and carrots, chopped
- 1 cup white wine
- A pinch of black pepper

Instructions:
1. Heat up a pan with half of the oil over medium high heat, add onion, stir; cook for 10 minutes and transfer to a baking dish.
2. Add the rest of the oil to the pan and heat up again over medium heat.
3. Add squash, stir and cook for 10 minutes more.
4. Add garlic, stir and cook for 2 minutes.
5. Add stock, wine and a pinch of black pepper, stir; cook for 10 minutes more, transfer to a blender and pulse really well.
6. Spread this over sautéed onions from the baking dish, also add mixed veggies, toss a bit, place in the oven at 400 °F and bake for 1 hour. Divide between plates and serve warm as a side dish.

Nutrition Facts Per Serving: Calories: 230; Fat: 4; Fiber: 4; Carbs: 6; Protein: 12

Grilled Artichokes

(Prep + Cook Time: 40 minutes | **Servings**: 4)

Ingredients:
- Juice of 1 lemon
- A pinch of sea salt
- Black pepper to the taste
- 2 artichokes; trimmed and cut into halves lengthwise
- 4 garlic cloves; chopped
- 3/4 cup extra virgin olive oil

Instructions:
1. Put water in a bowl; add half of the lemon juice and artichoke halves and leave aside for now.
2. Put water in a bowl; place on stove over medium high heat, bring to a boil, add artichokes, cook for 15 minutes and drain them.
3. Put artichokes in a bowl; add the rest of the lemon juice, the oil, a pinch of salt, black pepper to the taste and garlic and toss to coat.
4. Drain artichokes and reserve lemon dressing, arrange them on preheated grill over medium-high heat, grill them for 10 minutes and transfer them to a plate. Serve as a side dish with the reserved dressing drizzled on top.

Nutrition Facts Per Serving: Calories: 119; Fat: 3.8; Carbs: 23; Fiber: 11.4; Protein: 6.1

Pumpkin Salad

(**Prep + Cook Time**: 40 minutes | **Servings**: 6)

Ingredients:
- 1 tbsp. honey + 2 tsp. honey
- 2 tbsp. olive oil + 2 tsp. olive oil
- 21 oz. pumpkin; peeled, seeded and cut into medium pieces
- 2 tsp. sesame seeds
- 1 tbsp. lemon juice
- 2 tsp. mustard
- 4 oz. baby spinach

- 2 tbsp. pine nuts; toasted
- A pinch of sea salt
- Black pepper to the taste

Instructions:

1. In a bowl; mix pumpkin with a pinch of salt, black pepper, 2 tsp. oil and 2 tsp. honey, toss to coat well, spread on a lined baking sheet, place in the oven at 400 °F and bake for 25 minutes.
2. Leave pumpkin pieces to cool down a bit, add sesame seeds, toss to coat, place in the oven again and bake for 5 minutes more.
3. In a bowl; mix lemon juice with 1 tbsp. honey, 2 tbsp. oil and mustard and stir well.
4. Leave pumpkin to completely cool down and transfer it to a salad bowl.
5. Add baby spinach and pine nuts and stir. Add salad dressing you've made, toss to coat well, divide between plates and serve as a side salad.

Nutrition Facts Per Serving: Calories: 220; Fat: 10; Fiber: 2; Carbs: 7; Protein: 6

Fennel Side Dish

(**Prep + Cook Time:** 10 minutes | **Servings:** 4)

Ingredients:

- 3 tbsp. lemon juice
- 1 lb. fennel; chopped
- A pinch of sea salt
- 2 tbsp. olive oil
- A pinch of black pepper

Instructions:

1. In a salad bowl; mix fennel with a pinch of salt and black pepper and stir.
2. In another bowl; mix oil with a pinch of salt, pepper and lemon juice and whisk well.

3. Add this to the salad bowl; toss to coat well and divide between plates. Serve as a Paleo side.

Nutrition Facts Per Serving: Calories: 100; Fat: 1; Fiber: 1; Carbs: 1; Protein: 3

Butternut Squash Side Dish

(**Prep + Cook Time**: 50 minutes | **Servings**: 4)

Ingredients:
- 2 tbsp. coconut oil
- 1 butternut squash; peeled and chopped
- 3 garlic cloves; finely minced
- 1 tbsp. thyme; chopped
- A pinch of sea salt
- Black pepper to the taste

Instructions:
1. Heat up a pan with the oil over medium-high heat, add garlic, squash and thyme, stir and cook for 5-6 minutes.
2. Spread well in the pan and cook for another 5 minutes. Reduce heat, cover pan and cook for 10 more minutes, stirring from time to time.
3. Add a pinch of salt and pepper to the taste, stir again, take off heat, transfer to plates and serve as a side dish.

Nutrition Facts Per Serving: Calories: 83; Fat: 2.4; Carbs: 16; Fiber: 3; Sugar: 3; Protein: 1.4

Poached Kohlrabi Dish

(**Prep + Cook Time**: 27 minutes | **Servings**: 3)

Ingredients:
- 4 tbsp. ghee
- 3 kohlrabi; peeled and cubed
- 1 tbsp. sage; chopped
- A pinch of sea salt and black pepper

Instructions:

1. Heat up a pan with the ghee over medium high heat, add kohlrabi, a pinch of salt and black pepper, stir and cook for 15 minutes.
2. Add sage, stir again, cook for 2 minutes more, divide between plates and serve.

Nutrition Facts Per Serving: Calories: 120; Fat: 2; Fiber: 1; Carbs: 2; Protein: 5

Mashed Carrots

(**Prep + Cook Time**: 26 minutes | **Servings**: 4)

Ingredients:
- 1 lb. rutabaga; peeled and chopped
- A pinch of sea salt
- Black pepper to the taste
- 4 tbsp. ghee
- 1 lb. carrots; chopped
- 1 tbsp. parsley; chopped

Instructions:
1. Put rutabaga and carrots in a pot, add water to cover, place on stove, bring to a boil over medium-high heat, reduce temperature, cover pot and cook for 20 minutes.
2. Drain carrots and rutabaga, transfer them to a bowl; mash with a potato masher, mix with ghee, a pinch of salt and pepper to the taste, stir well and divide among plates. Sprinkle parsley on top and serve as a side dish.

Nutrition Facts Per Serving: Calories: 100; Fat: 1; Carbs: 11; Fiber: 3.5; Sugar: 3; Fiber: 1.4

Chard Side Dish

(**Prep + Cook Time**: 20 minutes | **Servings**: 2)

Ingredients:
- **1/2 cup cashews; chopped**
- **1 bunch chard; cut into thin strips**

- **A pinch of sea salt**
- **Black pepper to the taste**
- 1 tbsp. coconut oil

Instructions:

1. Heat up a pan with the oil over medium heat, add chard and cashews, stir and cook for 10 minutes.
2. Add a pinch of salt and pepper to the taste, stir; cook for 1 minute more, take off heat, transfer to plates and serve as a side dish.

Nutrition Facts Per Serving: Calories: 60; Fat: 0.3; Carbs: 2; Fiber: 1; Protein: 2; Sugar: 0

Special Paleo Side Salad

(**Prep + Cook Time**: 10 minutes | **Servings**: 2)

Ingredients:

- 2 cups arugula
- 1 tbsp. olive oil
- 1 tbsp. balsamic vinegar
- 2 cups kale; torn
- 3 tbsp. red onion; chopped
- 4 kumquats; sliced
- 1 small avocado; pitted, peeled and cubed
- 3 figs; chopped
- 1/2 cup walnuts; chopped

Instructions:

1. In a bowl; mix vinegar with the oil, whisk well and leave aside for now.
2. In a salad bowl; mix arugula with kale, onion, kumquats, avocado, figs and walnuts and stir. Add salad dressing, toss to coat and serve.

Nutrition Facts Per Serving: Calories: 100; Fat: 1; Fiber: 0; Carbs: 0; Protein: 4

Roasted Brussels Sprouts

(**Prep + Cook Time**: 40 minutes | **Servings**: 6)

Ingredients:

- 1½ lbs. Brussels sprouts; cut in halves
- A pinch of sea salt
- Black pepper to the taste
- 1 tsp. garlic powder
- 2/3 cups pecans; chopped
- 1 cup pomegranate seeds
- 2 tbsp. extra virgin olive oil

Instructions:

1. In a bowl; mix oil with a pinch of sea salt, pepper and garlic powder and stir well.
2. Add Brussels sprouts and pecans and toss to coat. Spread this in lined baking dish, introduce in the oven at 400 °F and bake for 30 minutes.
3. Take sprouts out of the oven, transfer to plates, top with pomegranate seeds and serve as a side dish.

Nutrition Facts Per Serving: Calories: 100; Fat: 1; Carbs: 10; Fiber: 4; Sugar: 1; Protein: 4

Pumpkin And Bok Choy

(**Prep + Cook Time**: 25 minutes | **Servings**: 4)

Ingredients:

- 2 tsp. sesame oil
- 2 tbsp. olive oil
- 3 tbsp. coconut aminos
- 1 inch ginger; grated
- A pinch of red pepper flakes
- 4 bok choy heads; cut in quarters
- 2 garlic cloves; minced
- 1 small pumpkin; peeled, seeded and thinly sliced
- 1 tbsp. sesame seeds; toasted

Instructions:

1. Heat up a pan with the sesame and olive oil over medium heat, add coconut aminos, garlic, pepper flakes and ginger, stir; cook for 1 minute and take off heat.
2. Heat up another pan, add some water, bring to a simmer over medium high heat, add pumpkin pieces, cover and cook them for 10 minutes.
3. Drain pumpkin slices really well and transfer them to a platter.
4. Add bok choy to the pan with the water, heat it up again over medium high heat, cover and cook for 5 minutes.
5. Drain this as well and add to the same platter with the pumpkin. Add sesame oil mix from the pan, add sesame seeds as well, toss everything and serve as a side dish.

Nutrition Facts Per Serving: Calories: 160; Fat: 2; Fiber: 2; Carbs: 4; Protein: 5

Mashed Sweet Potatoes

(**Prep + Cook Time**: 1 hour 25 minutes | **Servings**: 6)

Ingredients:
- 1/4 cup coconut oil
- 3 lbs. sweet potatoes
- A pinch of sea salt
- Black pepper to the taste

Instructions:
1. Wash sweet potatoes and arrange them on a lined baking sheet.
2. Place in the oven at 375 °F and bake them for 1 hour.
3. Leave potatoes to cool down, peel and transfer flesh to a baking dish.
4. Mash them well, add oil and stir very well.
5. Also, add a pinch of salt and black pepper to the taste, stir well again and bake in the oven at 375 °F for 15 minutes more. Divide between plates and serve as a side dish.

Nutrition Facts Per Serving: Calories: 240; Fat: 1; Fiber: 4; Carbs: 6; Protein: 4

Tasty Butternut Squash

(**Prep + Cook Time**: 45 minutes | **Servings**: 6)

Ingredients:

- 2 tbsp. coconut oil; melted
- 2 lbs. butternut squash; peeled, seeded and cubed
- 2 tsp. thyme; chopped
- A pinch of black pepper

Instructions:

1. In a bowl; mix squash cubes with oil, thyme and pepper and toss to coat well.
2. Spread this on a lined baking sheet, place in the oven at 425 °F and bake for 35 minutes, stirring every once in a while.
3. Leave roasted squash pieces to cool down, divide between plates and serve as a Paleo side.

Nutrition Facts Per Serving: Calories: 100; Fat: 1; Fiber: 2; Carbs: 3; Protein: 6

Mushrooms And Thyme Side Dish

(**Prep + Cook Time**: 35 minutes | **Servings**: 4)

Ingredients:

- 4 garlic cloves; finely chopped
- 2 tbsp. extra virgin olive oil
- 8 thyme springs
- 16 oz. mushrooms
- A pinch of sea salt
- White pepper to the taste

Instructions:

1. Grease a baking dish with some of the oil and spread thyme on the bottom.

2. Add mushrooms, garlic, season them with a pinch of salt and pepper to the taste and drizzle the rest of the olive oil all over.
3. Introduce dish in the oven at 375 °F and bake for 25 minutes. Take mushrooms out of the oven, divide between plates, pour pan sauces over them and serve as a side dish.

Nutrition Facts Per Serving: Calories: 131; Fat: 7; Carbs: 10; Fiber: 3; Sugar: 2. protein 8.1

Tasty Creamy Mashed Pumpkin

(**Prep + Cook Time**: 55 minutes | **Servings**: 4)

Ingredients:
- 1 tsp. cinnamon powder
- 1 cup unsweetened coconut; shredded
- 1 pumpkin; peeled, seeded and cubed
- 1/2 cup coconut oil
- A pinch of white pepper
- A pinch of sea salt

Instructions:
1. Put water in a pot, add pumpkin cubes, heat up over medium high heat, cover and cook for 30 minutes.
2. Drain water, add a pinch of salt and pepper, oil and coconut to the pan, stir and cook everything for 3 minutes more.
3. Mash using a potato masher, add cinnamon, stir well, cook for 2 minutes more, divide between plates and serve.

Nutrition Facts Per Serving: Calories: 100; Fat: 2; Fiber: 2; Carbs: 3; Protein: 3

Eggplant And Mushrooms

(**Prep + Cook Time**: 1 hour 40 minutes | **Servings**: 4)

Ingredients:
- **2 lbs. oyster mushrooms; chopped**
- **6 oz. bacon; chopped**
- **1 yellow onion; chopped**

- **2 eggplants; cubed**
- **3 celery stalks; chopped**
- **1 tbsp. parsley; chopped**
- **A pinch of sea salt**
- **Black pepper to the taste**
- **1 tbsp. savory; dried**
- 3 tbsp. coconut oil

Instructions:
1. Put eggplant pieces in a bowl; add a pinch of salt and black pepper, toss a bit, leave aside for 1 hour, drain well and leave aside in a bowl.
2. Heat up a pan with the oil over medium high heat, add onion, stir and cook for 4 minutes.
3. Add bacon, stir and cook for 4 more minutes.
4. Add eggplant pieces, mushrooms, celery, savory and black pepper to the taste, stir and cook for 15 minutes. Add parsley, stir again, cook for a couple more minutes, divide between plates and serve.

Nutrition Facts Per Serving: Calories: 200; Fat: 3; Fiber: 3; Carbs: 6; Protein: 9

Paleo Plantain Fries

(**Prep + Cook Time**: 20 minutes | **Servings**: 4)

Ingredients:
- 1/2 cup duck fat
- 2 green plantains; peeled and sliced
- A pinch of sea salt
- Black pepper to the taste

Instructions:
1. Heat up a pan with the duck fat over medium high heat, season plantain slices with a pinch of salt and black pepper, add half of them to the pan, cook for 5 minutes and transfer to paper towels.

2. Fry the second batch of plantain slices, drain grease as well, divide them between plates and serve them as a side.

Nutrition Facts Per Serving: Calories: 120; Fat: 2; Fiber: 2; Carbs: 4; Protein: 3

Stuffed Artichokes

(**Prep + Cook Time**: 1 hour 20 minutes | **Servings**: 4)

Ingredients:

- 4 artichokes; stems cut off and hearts chopped
- 3 garlic cloves; minced
- 2 cups spinach; chopped
- 1 tbsp. coconut oil
- 1 yellow onion; chopped
- 4 oz. bacon; chopped, cooked and crumbled
- A pinch of black pepper

Instructions:

1. Put artichokes in a pot, add water to cover, bring to a boil over medium heat, cook for 30 minutes, drain them and leave them aside to cool down.
2. Heat up a pan with the oil over medium high heat, add onion, stir and cook for 10 minutes.
3. Add spinach, stir; cook for 3 minutes, take off heat and leave aside to cool down.
4. Put cooked bacon in your food processor, add artichoke insides as well and pulse really well.
5. Add this to spinach and onion mix and stir well everything.
6. Place artichoke cups on a lined baking sheet, stuff them with spinach mix, place in the oven at 375 °F and bake for 30 minutes. Arrange them on plates and serve as a side with a juicy steak.

Nutrition Facts Per Serving: Calories: 200; Fat: 3; Fiber: 2; Carbs: 6; Protein: 8

Plantain Mash

(**Prep + Cook Time**: 40 minutes | **Servings**: 4)

Ingredients:

- 6 oz. bacon; chopped
- 3 green bananas; peeled, cut in halves lengthwise and cut in semi-circles
- 4 garlic cloves; minced
- 1 yellow onion; chopped
- 2 tbsp. coconut oil
- A pinch of sea salt

Instructions:

1. Put water in a pot, bring to a boil over medium high heat, add plantain slices, cover and cook them for 20 minutes.
2. Drain plantains and leave them aside for now.
3. Heat up a pan over medium high heat, add bacon, stir and cook for 5 minutes.
4. Add garlic and onion, stir; cook for 5 minutes more, drain excess grease and transfer everything to a blender.
5. Add plantains and 2 tbsp. oil and pulse really well. Add a pinch of sea salt, blend again, divide between plates and serve.

Nutrition Facts Per Serving: Calories: 200; Fat: 1; Fiber: 4; Carbs: 6; Protein: 2

Paleo Roasted Broccoli

(**Prep + Cook Time**: 40 minutes | **Servings**: 4)

Ingredients:

- 8 garlic cloves; minced
- 1/4 cup avocado oil
- 8 cups broccoli florets
- Zest from 1 lemon; grated
- 1/4 cup parsley; chopped
- Black pepper to the taste

124

- A pinch of sea salt

Instructions:

1. In a bowl; mix broccoli with salt, pepper, oil, garlic and lemon zest, toss to coat, spread on a lined baking sheet, place in the oven at 450 °F and bake for 30 minutes.
2. Take baked broccoli out of the oven, divide between plates, sprinkle parsley on top and serve as a side.

Nutrition Facts Per Serving: Calories: 120; Fat: 1; Fiber: 2; Carbs: 3; Protein: 6

Amazing Paleo Side Dish

(**Prep + Cook Time**: 1 hour 10 minutes | **Servings**: 4)

Ingredients:

- 6 cups cauliflower florets
- 1½ lbs. turnips; thinly sliced
- 1 egg
- 2 cups chicken stock
- 1/4 cup avocado oil
- A pinch of sea salt
- Black pepper to the taste

Instructions:

1. Put stock in a pot, bring to a simmer over medium high heat, add cauliflower, stir; cover and cook for 15 minutes.
2. Transfer this to your food processor and blend well.
3. Add oil and blend well again.
4. In a bowl; whisk the egg with 1 tbsp. of the cauliflower mix.
5. Add this to cauliflower and pulse again well.
6. Add a pinch of salt and pepper and stir again.
7. Arrange turnips slices into a baking dish, pour the cauliflower purée over them, place in the oven at 375 °F and bake for 30 minutes. Divide between plates and serve.

Nutrition Facts Per Serving: Calories: 230; Fat: 3; Fiber: 2; Carbs: 4; Protein: 6

Broccoli And Tasty Hazelnuts

(**Prep + Cook Time**: 25 minutes | **Servings**: 4)

Ingredients:
- 1 tbsp. olive oil
- 1 garlic clove; minced
- 1 lb. broccoli florets
- 1/3 cup hazelnuts
- Black pepper to the taste

Instructions:
1. Heat up a pan with the oil over medium high heat, add hazelnuts, stir and cook for 5 minutes.
2. Transfer hazelnuts to a bowl and leave them aside for now.
3. Heat up the same pan again over medium high heat, add broccoli and garlic, stir; cover and cook for 6 minutes more. Add hazelnuts and black pepper to the taste, stir; divide between plates and serve.

Nutrition Facts Per Serving: Calories: 130; Fat: 3; Fiber: 2; Carbs: 5; Protein: 6

Roasted Green Beans

(**Prep + Cook Time**: 30 minutes | **Servings**: 4)

Ingredients:
- 1½ lbs. green beans
- 2 tbsp. lemon juice
- A pinch of sea salt
- 3 tbsp. avocado oil

Instructions:
1. In a bowl; mix green beans with a pinch of salt, oil and lemon juice, toss to coat well, spread on a lined baking sheet, place in the oven at 450 °F and roast for 20 minutes.
2. Leave green beans to cool down a bit, divide them between plates and serve.

Nutrition Facts Per Serving: Calories: 100; Fat: 3; Fiber: 1; Carbs: 4; Protein: 9

Paleo Tapioca Root Fries

(**Prep + Cook Time**: 1 hour 10 minutes | **Servings**: 4)

Ingredients:
- 2½ lb. tapioca root; cut in medium fries
- 1/2 cup duck fat; soft
- Black pepper to the taste
- A pinch of smoked paprika

Instructions:
1. Put some water in a pot and bring to a boil over medium high heat. Add tapioca fries, boil for 10 minutes and drain them well.
2. Spread them on a lined baking sheet, add black pepper, paprika and duck fat, toss everything to coat well, place in the oven at 375 °F and bake for 45 minutes.
3. Leave your tapioca fries to cool down a bit, divide them between plates and serve as a side.

Nutrition Facts Per Serving: Calories: 120; Fat: 2; Fiber: 2; Carbs: 4; Protein: 10

Stir Fried Side Dish

(**Prep + Cook Time**: 25 minutes | **Servings**: 4)

Ingredients:
- 1 tsp. ginger; grated
- 1 lb. white mushrooms; sliced
- 1 bunch turnip greens; trimmed
- 2 garlic cloves; minced
- Black pepper to the taste
- A pinch of sea salt
- 1/2 cup raw almonds
- 1/4 cup lime juice

- 2 tbsp. coconut oil; melted
- 1 tbsp. coconut aminos
- 2 tsp. arrowroot flour

Instructions:
1. Heat up a pan with the oil over medium high heat, add mushrooms and turnips greens, stir and cook for 2 minutes.
2. Add ginger and garlic, stir and cook for 2 minutes more.
3. Add lime juice, almonds, arrowroot, coconut aminos, a pinch of salt and black pepper, stir and cook for 10 minutes more. Stir your mix again, divide it between plates and serve.

Nutrition Facts Per Serving: Calories: 120; Fat: 2; Fiber: 2; Carbs: 4; Protein: 5

Brussels Sprouts Side Dish

(Prep + Cook Time: 40 minutes | **Servings:** 4)

Ingredients:
- 1/4 cup avocado oil
- 4 lbs. Brussels sprouts; cut in quarters
- A pinch of sea salt
- Black pepper to the taste

Instructions:
1. In a bowl; mix Brussels sprouts with oil, salt and pepper, toss to coat well, spread on a lined baking sheet, place in the oven at 375 °F and bake for 30 minutes.
2. Divide between plates and serve as a Paleo side dish!

Nutrition Facts Per Serving: Calories: 120; Fat: 1; Fiber: 1; Carbs: 2; Protein: 5

Turnips And Sauce

(Prep + Cook Time: 25 minutes | **Servings:** 4)

Ingredients:
- 1 tbsp. lemon juice
- Zest from 2 oranges
- 16 oz. turnips; thinly sliced

128

- 3 tbsp. coconut oil
- 1 tbsp. rosemary; chopped
- A pinch of sea salt
- Black pepper to the taste

Instructions:
1. Heat up a pan with the oil over medium high heat, add turnips, stir and cook for 4 minutes.
2. Add lemon juice, a pinch of salt, black pepper and rosemary, stir and cook for 10 minutes more. Take off heat, add orange zest, stir; divide between plates and serve.

Nutrition Facts Per Serving: Calories: 90; Fat: 1; Fiber: 2; Carbs: 3; Protein: 4

Paleo Taro Dish

(**Prep + Cook Time**: 35 minutes | **Servings**: 4)

Ingredients:
- 2 tsp. rosemary; dried
- 2 lbs. taro
- 3 tbsp. coconut oil
- 1/2 tsp. garlic powder
- A pinch of sea salt
- Black pepper to the taste

Instructions:
1. Put taro in a steamer, steam for 15 minutes, leave them to cool down, peel them and cut into quarters.
2. Heat up a pan with the oil over medium high heat, add taro, rosemary, garlic powder, salt and pepper, toss to coat and place in preheated broiler.
3. Broil for 10 minutes, divide between plates and serve as a Paleo side dish.

Nutrition Facts Per Serving: Calories: 120; Fat: 3; Fiber: 2; Carbs: 4; Protein: 7

Roasted Cauliflower

(Prep + Cook Time: 40 minutes | **Servings**: 4)

Ingredients:
- 1 cauliflower head; florets separated
- 1/4 cup coconut oil; melted
- 1/4 cup parsley; chopped
- 2 tsp. lemon zest; grated
- A pinch of sea salt and black pepper
- 10 garlic cloves; minced

Instructions:
1. Spread cauliflower florets on a lined baking sheet, add oil and toss to coat.
2. Add a pinch of salt and black pepper, garlic and lemon zest, toss again to coat well, place in the oven at 450 °F and bake for 30 minutes.
3. Take cauliflower out of the oven, sprinkle parsley on top, stir gently, divide between plates and serve.

Nutrition Facts Per Serving: Calories: 100; Fat: 1; Fiber: 2; Carbs: 4; Protein: 12

Mushrooms And Red Chard Side Dish

(Prep + Cook Time: 25 minutes | **Servings**: 4)

Ingredients:
- 1/2 lb. brown mushrooms; sliced
- 5 cups kale; roughly chopped
- 1½ tbsp. coconut oil
- 3 cups red chard; chopped
- 2 tbsp. water
- Black pepper to the taste

Instructions:
1. Heat up a pan with the oil over medium high heat, add mushrooms, stir and cook for 5 minutes.
2. Add red chard, kale and water, stir and cook for 10 minutes.

3. Add black pepper to the taste, stir and cook for a couple more minutes. Divide between plates and serve.

Nutrition Facts Per Serving: Calories: 100; Fat: 1; Fiber: 1; Carbs: 5; Protein: 3

Butternut Squash Mix

(**Prep + Cook Time**: 40 minutes | **Servings**: 4)

Ingredients:
- 1/2 tsp. cinnamon powder
- 2 tbsp. red palm oil
- 2 apples; peeled, cored and cubed
- 1 green plantain; peeled and cubed
- 1½ lbs. butternut squash; peeled, seeded and cubed

Instructions:
1. In a baking dish, mix apples with plantain, squash, cinnamon and oil, toss to coat, place in the oven at 350 °F and roast for 30 minutes.
2. Leave this mix to cool down a bit before dividing on plates and serving.

Nutrition Facts Per Serving: Calories: 100; Fat: 2; Fiber: 2; Carbs: 4; Protein: 10

Spaghetti Squash

(**Prep + Cook Time**: 65 minutes | **Servings**: 4)

Ingredients:
- 1 spaghetti squash; cut in halves and seeded
- 12 sage leaves
- 3 tbsp. ghee
- A pinch of sea salt
- Black pepper to the taste

Instructions:
1. Place spaghetti squash on a lined baking sheet, place in the oven at 375 °F and bake for 40 minutes.

2. Take spaghetti squash out of the oven and scoop strings of flesh.
3. Heat up a pan with the ghee over medium heat, add sage, cook for 5 minutes and transfer them to paper towels.
4. Heat up the pan again over medium heat, add spaghetti squash, a pinch of sea salt and black pepper to the taste, stir and cook for 3 minutes. Crumble sage leaves, add them to spaghetti, stir; divide between plates and serve as a side.

Nutrition Facts Per Serving: Calories: 100; Fat: 6; Fiber: 2; Carbs: 6; Protein: 2

Squash And Cranberries

(**Prep + Cook Time**: 40 minutes | **Servings**: 2)

Ingredients:
- 1 tbsp. coconut oil
- 1 butternut squash; peeled and cubed
- 2 garlic cloves; minced
- 1 small yellow onion; chopped
- 12 oz. canned coconut milk
- 1 tsp. curry powder
- 1 tsp. cinnamon powder
- 1/2 cup cranberries

Instructions:
1. Spread squash pieces on a lined baking sheet, place in the oven at 425 °F and bake for 15 minutes.
2. Take squash out of the oven and leave aside for now.
3. Heat up a pan with the oil over medium high heat, add garlic and onion, stir and cook for 5 minutes.
4. Add roasted squash, stir and cook for 3 minutes.
5. Add coconut milk, cranberries, cinnamon and curry powder, stir and cook for 5 minutes more. Divide between plates and serve as a side dish!

Nutrition Facts Per Serving: Calories: 100; Fat: 2; Fiber: 4; Carbs: 8; Protein: 2

Kale And Beets

(Prep + Cook Time: 40 minutes | **Servings**: 4)

Ingredients:
- 1 tbsp. coconut oil
- 4 cups kale; torn
- 3 beets; cut into quarters and thinly sliced
- 2 tbsp. water
- A pinch of cayenne pepper

Instructions:
1. Put water in a pot, add beets, bring to a boil over medium high heat, cover, reduce temperature, cook for 20 minutes and drain.
2. Heat up a pan with the oil over medium high heat, add kale and the water, stir and cook for 10 minutes.
3. Add beets and cayenne pepper, stir; cook for 2 minutes more, divide between plates and serve as a side dish!

Nutrition Facts Per Serving: Calories: 120; Fat: 2; Fiber: 1; Carbs: 2; Protein: 4

Paleo Kale Dish

(Prep + Cook Time: 30 minutes | **Servings**: 4)

Ingredients:
- 2 celery stalks; chopped
- 5 cups kale; torn
- 1 small red bell pepper; chopped
- 3 tbsp. water
- 1 tbsp. coconut oil

Instructions:
1. Heat up a pan with the oil over medium high heat, add celery, stir and cook for 10 minutes.
2. Add kale, water and bell pepper, stir and cook for 10 minutes more. Divide between plates and serve really soon!

Nutrition Facts Per Serving: Calories: 90; Fat: 1; Fiber: 2; Carbs: 2; Protein: 6

Cauliflower And Leeks

(**Prep + Cook Time**: 30 minutes | **Servings**: 4)

Ingredients:
- 1½ cups leeks; chopped
- 1½ cups cauliflower florets
- 2 garlic cloves; minced
- 1½ cups artichoke hearts
- 2 tbsp. bacon grease
- Black pepper to the taste

Instructions:
1. Heat up a pan with the bacon grease over medium high heat, add garlic, leeks, cauliflower florets and artichoke hearts, stir and cook for 20 minutes. Add black pepper, stir; divide between plates and serve.

Nutrition Facts Per Serving: Calories: 110; Fat: 2; Fiber: 2; Carbs: 6; Protein: 3

Braised Cabbage Side Dish

(**Prep + Cook Time**: 30 minutes | **Servings**: 4)

Ingredients:
- 1 small cabbage head; shredded
- 2 tbsp. water
- 6 oz. bacon; chopped
- A pinch of black pepper
- A pinch of sweet paprika
- 1 tbsp. dill; chopped

Instructions:
1. Put bacon in a pan and heat up over medium high heat.
2. Stir and cook for 8 minutes.
3. Add cabbage and 1 tbsp. water, stir and cook for 5 minutes.
4. Add the rest of the water, black pepper, paprika and dill, stir and cook for 5 minutes more. Divide between plates and serve as a side dish!

Nutrition Facts Per Serving: Calories: 90; Fat: 2; Fiber: 2; Carbs: 8; Protein: 6

Mint Zucchini

(Prep + Cook Time: 17 minutes | **Servings**: 4)

Ingredients:

- 2 tbsp. mint
- 2 zucchinis; cut into halves and then slice into half moons
- 1 tbsp. coconut oil
- 1/2 tbsp. dill; chopped
- A pinch of cayenne pepper

Instructions:

1. Heat up a pan with the oil over medium high heat, add zucchinis, stir and cook for 6 minutes.
2. Add cayenne, dill and mint, stir; cook for 1 minute more, divide between plates and serve.

Nutrition Facts Per Serving: Calories: 80; Fat: 0; Fiber: 1; Carbs: 1; Protein: 5

Paleo Basil Zucchini Spaghetti

(Prep + Cook Time: 1 hour 20 minutes | **Servings**: 4)

Ingredients:

- 1/3 cup bacon grease
- 4 zucchinis; cut with a spiralizer
- 1/4 cup basil; chopped
- A pinch of sea salt
- Black pepper to the taste
- 1/2 cup walnuts; chopped
- 2 garlic cloves; minced

Instructions:

1. In a bowl; mix zucchini spaghetti with a pinch of salt and pepper, toss to coat, leave aside for 1 hour, drain well, rinse, drain again and put in a bowl.
2. Heat up a pan with the bacon grease over medium high heat, add zucchini spaghetti and garlic, stir and cook for 5 minutes.

3. Add basil and walnuts and some black pepper, stir and cook for 3 minutes more. Divide between plates and serve.

Nutrition Facts Per Serving: Calories: 240; Fat: 1; Fiber: 4; Carbs: 7; Protein: 13

Spicy Sweet Potatoes

(**Prep + Cook Time**: 50 minutes | **Servings**: 4)

Ingredients:
- 4 sweet potatoes; peeled and thinly sliced
- 2 tsp. nutmeg
- 2 tbsp. coconut oil; melted
- Cayenne pepper to the taste

Instructions:
1. In a bowl; mix sweet potato slices with nutmeg, cayenne and oil and toss to coat really well.
2. Spread these on a lined baking sheet, place in the oven at 350 °F and bake for 25 minutes.
3. Take potatoes out of the oven, flip them, put them back into the oven and bake for 15 minutes more. Serve as a tasty Paleo side dish!

Nutrition Facts Per Serving: Calories: 140; Fat: 3; Fiber: 2; Carbs: 4; Protein: 10

Paleo Dill Carrots

(**Prep + Cook Time**: 40 minutes | **Servings**: 4)

Ingredients:
- 1 tbsp. coconut oil; melted
- 2 tbsp. dill; chopped
- 1 lb. baby carrots
- 1 tbsp. honey
- A pinch of black pepper

Instructions:
1. Put carrots in a pot, add water to cover, bring to a boil over medium high heat, cover and simmer for 30 minutes.

2. Drain well, put carrots in a bowl; add melted oil, black pepper, dill and honey, stir very well, divide between plates and serve.

Nutrition Facts Per Serving: Calories: 120; Fat: 2; Fiber: 3; Carbs: 5; Protein: 6

Soups & Stews Recipes

Special Paleo Soup

(**Prep + Cook Time**: 55 minutes | **Servings**: 6)

Ingredients:
- 1 yellow onion; finely chopped
- 1 tbsp. avocado oil
- 3 thyme springs; chopped
- 3 garlic cloves; finely minced
- 28 oz. canned tomatoes; chopped
- 6 oz. tomato paste
- 1/4 cup water
- 1 lb. sausage; chopped
- 14 oz. beef stock
- 6 mushrooms; chopped
- 1 small red bell pepper; chopped
- 5 oz. pepperoni
- 2.5 oz. black olives; chopped
- A pinch of red pepper flakes

Instructions:
1. Heat up a pot with the oil over medium high heat and melt it.
2. Add half of the onion, garlic and thyme, stir and cook for 5 minutes.
3. Add tomatoes, tomato paste and water, stir; bring to a boil, reduce heat to medium-low and simmer for 20 minutes.
4. Pour this into your blender, pulse well and leave aside for now.

5. Heat up a pot over medium-high heat, add sausage, stir and cook for a few minutes, breaking into small pieces with a fork.
6. Add the rest of the onion, mushrooms and the bell pepper, stir and cook for 5 minutes.
7. Add tomato soup you've blended and beef stock, stir and cook for 5 more minutes.
8. Heat up a pan over medium high heat, add pepperoni slices, stir and cook until they brown. Pour soup into bowls, top with red pepper flakes, olives and pepperoni.

Nutrition Facts Per Serving: Calories: 224; Fat: 16; Carbs: 8; Fiber: 3; Sugar: 5.5; Protein: 7

Healthy Veggie Stew

(**Prep + Cook Time**: 1 hour 10 minutes | **Servings**: 6)

Ingredients:
- 4 lbs. mixed root vegetables (parsnips; carrots, rutabagas, beets, celery root, turnips), chopped
- 6 tbsp. extra virgin olive oil
- 1 garlic head; cloves separated and peeled
- 1/2 cup yellow onion; chopped
- Black pepper to the taste
- 28 oz. canned tomatoes; peeled and chopped
- 1 tbsp. tomato paste
- 2 cups kale leaves; torn
- 1 tsp. oregano; dried
- Tabasco sauce for serving

Instructions:
1. In a baking dish, mix all root vegetables with black pepper, half of the oil and garlic, toss to coat, introduce in the oven at 450 degrees G and roast them for 45 minutes.
2. Heat up a pot with the rest of the oil over medium-high heat, add onions and cook for 2-3 minutes stirring often.
3. Add tomato paste, stir and cook 1 more minute.

4. Add tomatoes and their liquid, some salt and pepper and the oregano, stir; bring to a simmer, reduce heat to low and cook until veggies become roasted.
5. Take root veggies out of the oven, add them to the pot and stir.
6. Add kale, stir and cook for 5 minutes. Add Tabasco sauce to the taste, stir; transfer to bowls and serve.

Nutrition Facts Per Serving: Calories: 150; Fat: 7; Carbs: 17.2; Fiber: 3.7; Sugar: 5; Protein: 2.4

Lemon And Garlic Soup

(**Prep + Cook Time**: 20 minutes | **Servings**: 4)

Ingredients:
- 6 cups shellfish stock
- 1 tbsp. garlic; finely minced
- 1 tbsp. coconut oil; melted
- 2 eggs
- 1/2 cup lemon juice
- A pinch of sea salt
- White pepper to the taste
- 1 tbsp. arrowroot powder
- Cilantro; finely chopped for serving

Instructions:
1. Heat up a pot with the oil over medium high heat, add garlic, stir and cook for 2 minutes.
2. Add stock but reserve 1/2 cup, stir and bring to a simmer.
3. Meanwhile; in a bowl, mix eggs with sea salt, pepper, reserved stock, lemon juice and arrowroot and whisk very well.
4. Pour this into soup, stir and cook for a few minutes. Ladle into bowls and serve with chopped cilantro on top.

Nutrition Facts Per Serving: Calories: 135; Fat: 3; Carbs: 12; Fiber: 1; Protein: 8; Sugar: 0

Veggie Soup

(**Prep + Cook Time**: 55 minutes | **Servings**: 4)

Ingredients:

- 2 sweet potatoes; peeled and chopped
- 2 yellow onions; cut into eighths
- 2 lbs. carrots; diced
- 4 tbsp. coconut oil
- 1 head garlic; cloves peeled
- A pinch of sea salt
- Black pepper to the taste
- 2 cups chicken stock
- 3 tbsp. maple syrup

Instructions:

1. Put onions, carrots, sweet potatoes and garlic in a baking dish, add coconut oil, a pinch of sea salt and pepper to the taste, toss to coat, introduce in the oven at 425 °F and bake for 35 minutes.
2. Take veggies out of the oven, transfer to a pot, add chicken stock and heat everything up on the stove on medium-high heat.
3. Bring soup to a boil, reduce heat to medium, cover and simmer for 10 minutes. Transfer soup to your blender, add more pepper and the maple syrup, pulse well to obtain a cream, pour into soup bowls and serve.

Nutrition Facts Per Serving: Calories: 130; Fat: 3; Carbs: 12; Fiber: 3.5; Sugar: 6; Protein: 3

Chicken Soup

(**Prep + Cook Time**: 1 hour 15 minutes | **Servings**: 4)

Ingredients:

- 2 tsp. coconut oil
- 3 carrots; chopped
- 1 yellow onion; chopped
- 1 zucchini; chopped

- 12 oz. canned mushrooms; chopped
- 1/4 butternut squash; cubed
- 4 cups chicken meat; already cooked and shredded
- 2 tsp. rosemary; dried
- 1 tsp. thyme; dried
- 1 tbsp. apple cider vinegar
- 1 tsp. cumin
- 2½ cups chicken stock
- A pinch of sea salt
- Black pepper to the taste

Instructions:
1. Heat up a pot with the coconut oil over medium heat, add carrots and onion, stir and cook for 5 minutes.
2. Add zucchini, mushrooms and squash, stir and cook for 5 more minutes.
3. Add chicken meat, rosemary, thyme, vinegar, cumin and chicken stock.
4. Stir, bring to a boil, reduce heat to medium-low and simmer for 40 minutes. Add a pinch of salt and pepper to the taste, stir again, take off heat and pour into soup bowls.

Nutrition Facts Per Serving: Calories: 390; Fat: 2; Carbs: 34; Protein: 6; Sugar: 0; Fiber: 4

Simple Paleo Soup

(**Prep + Cook Time**: 10 minutes | **Servings**: 3)

Ingredients:
- 1 avocado; pitted and chopped
- 1 cucumber; chopped
- 2 bunches spinach
- 1½ cups watermelon; chopped
- 1 bunch cilantro; roughly chopped
- Juice from 2 lemons
- 1/2 cup coconut aminos

- 1/2 cup lime juice

Instructions:

1. In your kitchen blender, mix cucumber with avocado and pulse well.
2. Add cilantro, spinach and watermelon and blend again well.
3. Add lemon and lime juice and coconut amino and pulse a few more times. Transfer to soup bowls and enjoy!

Nutrition Facts Per Serving: Calories: 100; Fat: 7; Carbs: 6.5; Fiber: 3.5; Sugar: 2.4; Protein: 2.3

Delicious Tomato And Basil Soup

(**Prep + Cook Time**: 45 minutes | **Servings**: 4)

Ingredients:

- 56 oz. canned tomatoes; crushed
- 2 cups tomato juice
- 2 cups chicken stock
- 1/4 lb. coconut butter
- 14 basil leaves; torn
- 1 cup coconut milk
- Salt and black pepper to the taste

Instructions:

1. Put tomatoes, tomato juice and stock in a pot, heat up over medium-high heat, bring to a boil, reduce heat, stir and simmer for 30 minutes.
2. Pour this into your blender, add basil, pulse very well and return to pot.
3. Heat up soup again, add butter and coconut milk, stir and cook on low heat for a few more minutes. Add salt and pepper to the taste, stir well, pour into soup bowls and serve.

Nutrition Facts Per Serving: Calories: 170; Fat: 10; Carbs: 14; Protein: 2; Sugar: 1

Beef Soup

(**Prep + Cook Time**: 1 hour 10 minutes | **Servings**: 6)

Ingredients:

- 1 lb. organic beef; ground
- 1 lb. sausage; sliced
- 4 cups beef stock
- 30 oz. canned tomatoes; diced
- 1 green bell pepper; chopped
- 3 zucchinis; chopped
- 1 cup celery; chopped
- 1 tsp. Italian seasoning
- 1/2 yellow onion; chopped
- 1/2 tsp. oregano; dried
- 1/2 tsp. basil; dried
- 1/4 tsp. garlic powder
- A pinch of sea salt
- Black pepper to the taste

Instructions:

1. Heat up a pot over medium heat, add sausage and beef, stir; cook until it browns and drains excess fat.
2. Add tomatoes, zucchini, bell pepper, celery, onion, Italian seasoning, basil, oregano, garlic powder, sea salt, pepper to the taste and the stock.
3. stir; bring to a boil, reduce heat to medium-low and simmer for 1 hour. Pour into soup bowls and serve right away.

Nutrition Facts Per Serving: Calories: 370; Fat: 17; Carbs: 35; Fiber: 10; Protein: 25

French Chicken Stew

(**Prep + Cook Time**: 2 hours 15 minutes | **Servings**: 4)

Ingredients:

- 10 garlic cloves; peeled
- 30 black olives; pitted
- 2 lbs. chicken pieces

- 2 cups chicken stock
- 28 oz. canned tomatoes; chopped
- 2 tbsp. rosemary; chopped
- 2 tbsp. parsley leaves; chopped
- 2 tbsp. basil leaves; chopped
- A pinch of sea salt
- Black pepper to the taste
- A drizzle of extra virgin olive oil

Instructions:

1. Heat up a pot with some olive oil over medium-high heat, add chicken pieces, a pinch of sea salt and pepper to the taste and cook for 4 minutes, stirring often.
2. Add garlic, stir and brown for 2 minutes.
3. Add chicken stock, tomatoes, olives, thyme and rosemary, stir; cover pot and bake in the oven at 325 °F for 1 hour.
4. Add parsley and basil, stir; introduce in the oven again and bake for 45 more minutes. Leave stew to cool down for a few minutes, transfer to plates and serve.

Nutrition Facts Per Serving: Calories: 300; Fat: 48; Carbs: 16; Sugar: 0; Protein: 61

Beef And Plantain Stew

(**Prep + Cook Time**: 5 hours 10 minutes | **Servings**: 4)

Ingredients:

- 6 plantains; skinless and cubed
- 2 lbs. beef meat; cubed
- 3 cups collard greens; chopped
- A pinch of sea salt
- Black pepper to the taste
- 3 cups water
- 1/2 cup sweet paprika
- 3 tbsp. allspice
- 1/4 cup garlic powder

- 1 tsp. chili powder
- 1 tsp. cayenne pepper

Instructions:
1. In your slow cooker, mix beef with plantains, collard greens, water, paprika, garlic powder, allspice, chili powder, cayenne, a pinch of salt and pepper to the taste.
2. Stir, cover pot and cook on High for 5 hours. Uncover slow cooker, leave stew to cool down for a few minutes, transfer to bowls and serve.

Nutrition Facts Per Serving: Calories: 410; Fat: 11; Carbs: 39; Fiber: 10; Protein: 34; Sugar: 5

Delicious Beef Stew

(**Prep + Cook Time**: 2 hours 10 minutes | **Servings**: 4)

Ingredients:
- 2 lbs. beef fillet; cubed
- 1 red chili; seeded and chopped
- 1 brown onion; finely chopped
- 1 tsp. ghee
- 2 tbsp. extra virgin olive oil
- A pinch of sea salt
- Black pepper to the taste
- 2/3 tsp. nutmeg
- 2 tbsp. Worcestershire sauce; gluten free
- 1 garlic clove; minced
- 1/2 cup dried mushrooms
- 1/2 cup white wine
- 1/2 tbsp. dry sherry
- 1 tsp. rosemary; dry
- 4 thyme springs
- 1/4 tsp. fennel seeds
- 1-star anise
- 2 celery stick; chopped

- 2 carrots; thinly sliced
- 1-quart beef stock
- 6 button mushrooms; chopped
- 2 tbsp. almond flour
- 1 sweet potato; chopped

Instructions:

1. Heat up a pot with the ghee and the olive oil over medium-high heat, add onion, chili, some sea salt and pepper, stir and cook for 2-3 minutes.
2. Add meat, stir and brown it for 5 minutes.
3. Add Worcestershire sauce, wine, sherry, dried mushrooms, garlic, stock, thyme, fennel, rosemary, nutmeg and star anise, stir; bring to a boil, cover, reduce heat to low and cook for 1 hour and 10 minutes.
4. Add celery, carrots, fresh mushrooms, potato, stir; cover and cook for 15 minutes.
5. Increase heat to medium, uncover the pot and cook the stew for 15 minutes.
6. In a bowl; mix the flour with a cup of liquid from the stew, stir well, pour over stew and cook for 15 more minutes. Transfer to bowls and serve hot.

Nutrition Facts Per Serving: Calories: 313; Fat: 8; Carbs: 21; Fiber: 3; Sugar: 7; Protein: 38

Beef Stew

(**Prep + Cook Time**: 2 hours 10 minutes | **Servings**: 4)
Ingredients:
- 2 lbs. organic beef steak; cubed
- 1 tbsp. coconut oil
- A pinch of sea salt
- Black pepper to the taste
- 1 red chili pepper; chopped
- 1 yellow onion; chopped
- 1 tbsp. coconut aminos

- 1/2 cup white wine
- 1 tbsp. lemon juice
- A pinch of nutmeg; ground
- 2 garlic cloves; minced
- 1 tsp. thyme; dried
- 1/4 tsp. fennel seeds
- 1-star anise
- 1 tsp. rosemary; dried
- 4 cups beef stock
- 2 carrots; chopped
- 2 celery; sticks, chopped
- 1½ tbsp. arrowroot flour
- 1 sweet potato; chopped
- 6 white mushrooms; chopped

Instructions:

1. Heat up a pot with the oil over medium heat, add onion, stir and cook for 5 minutes.
2. Add a pinch of sea salt, black pepper to the taste and the chili pepper, stir and cook for 1-2 minutes more.
3. Add beef, stir and cook for 5 minutes.
4. Add coconut aminos, wine, lemon juice, garlic, thyme, rosemary, fennel, nutmeg, star anise and stock, stir and bring to a boil.
5. Cover the pot, cook for 1 hour and 15 minutes and then mix with celery, sweet potato, carrots and mushrooms.
6. Stir, cover pot again and cook for 10 minutes more.
7. Uncover pot, stir and cook everything for 15 minutes.
8. In a bowl; mix 2 tbsp. cooking liquid from the pot with the arrowroot flour and stir very well. Add this to the stew, stir; cook for a couple more minutes, divide into bowls and serve.

Nutrition Facts Per Serving: Calories: 313; Fat: 7; Fiber: 3; Carbs: 10; Protein: 23

Paleo Root Soup

(**Prep + Cook Time**: 1 hour 40 minutes | **Servings**: 8)

Ingredients:

- 1 sweet onion; chopped
- 2 tbsp. ghee
- 5 carrots; chopped
- 3 parsnips; chopped
- 3 beets; chopped
- 3 bacon slices
- 1-quart chicken stock
- A pinch of sea salt
- Black pepper to the taste
- 2 quarts water
- 1/2 tsp. chili flakes
- 1 tbsp. mixed thyme and rosemary

Instructions:

1. Heat up a Dutch oven with the ghee over medium-high heat, add onion, stir and cook for 5 minutes.
2. Add carrots, parsnips, beets, bacon, chicken stock and water and stir.
3. Also add sea salt, pepper to the taste, chili flakes, thyme and rosemary, stir again, bring to a boil, reduce heat to medium-low and simmer for 1 hour and 30 minutes. Pour into soup bowls and serve hot.

Nutrition Facts Per Serving: Calories: 180; Fat: 2; Carbs: 4; Fiber: 1; Sugar: 0.5; Protein: 3.5

Oxtail Stew

(**Prep + Cook Time**: 6 hours 15 minutes | **Servings**: 8)

Ingredients:

- 4½ lbs. oxtail; cut into medium chunks
- A drizzle of extra virgin olive oil
- 1 tbsp. extra virgin olive oil
- 2 leeks; chopped

- 4 carrots; chopped
- 2 celery sticks; chopped
- 4 thyme springs; chopped
- 4 rosemary springs; chopped
- 4 cloves
- 4 bay leaves
- Black pepper to the taste
- 2 tbsp. coconut flour
- 28 oz. canned plum tomatoes; chopped
- 9 oz. red wine
- 1-quart beef stock

Instructions:
1. In a roasting pan, mix oxtail with black pepper and a drizzle of oil.
2. Toss to coat, introduce in the oven at 425 °F and bake for 20 minutes.
3. Heat up a pot with 1 tbsp. oil over medium heat, add leeks, celery and carrots, stir and cook for 4 minutes.
4. Add thyme, rosemary and bay leaves, stir and cook everything for 20 minutes.
5. Take oxtail out of the oven and leave aside for a few minutes.
6. Add flour and cloves to veggies and stir.
7. Also add tomatoes, wine, oxtail and its juices and stock, stir; increase heat to high and bring to a boil.
8. Introduce pot in the oven at 325 °F and bake for 5 hours.
9. Take stew out of the oven, leave aside for 10 minutes, take oxtail out of the pot and discard bones. Return meat to pot, add more pepper to the taste, stir; transfer to plates and serve.

Nutrition Facts Per Serving: Calories: 523; Fat: 38; Carbs: 12; Sugar: 6.5; Fiber: 2.6; Protein: 28

Delightful Gazpacho

(**Prep + Cook Time**: 12 minutes | **Servings**: 4)

Ingredients:
- 8 tomatoes
- 1 red onion; chopped
- 1 cucumber; peeled and chopped
- 1 red bell pepper; chopped
- 1 green bell pepper; chopped
- 1 red chili pepper; chopped
- 3 garlic cloves
- 1 cup tomato juice
- 1 cup water
- 2 tbsp. apple cider vinegar
- Zest from 1/2 orange
- 3/4 cup olive oil
- A pinch of sea salt
- Black pepper to the taste

Instructions:
1. Put some water in a pot and bring to a boil over medium high heat.
2. Add tomatoes, leave them in boiling water for 2 minutes, drain and rinse them.
3. Peel, chop and put them in your food processor.
4. Add red onion, cucumber, red bell pepper, green bell pepper, chili pepper, garlic, tomato juice, water, vinegar, orange zest, olive oil, a pinch of salt and black pepper to the taste and pulse really well until you obtain cream. Ladle into soup bowls and serve cold.

Nutrition Facts Per Serving: Calories: 140; Fat: 1; Fiber: 1; Carbs: 3; Protein: 2

Awesome Chicken Stew

(**Prep + Cook Time**: 8 hours 15 minutes | **Servings**: 6)

Ingredients:
- 5 garlic cloves; finely chopped

- 2 celery stalks; chopped
- 2 yellow onions; chopped
- 2 carrots; chopped
- 30 oz. canned pumpkin puree
- 2 quarts chicken stock
- 2 cups chicken meat; chopped
- 1/4 cup coconut flour
- Black pepper to the taste
- 1/2 lb. baby spinach
- 1/4 tsp. cayenne pepper

Instructions:
1. In your slow cooker, mix chicken meat with onions, carrots, celery, garlic, pumpkin puree, chicken stock, black pepper, flour and cayenne, stir well, cover and cook on low for 7 hours and 50 minutes.
2. Uncover slow cooker, add spinach, cover again and cook for 10 more minutes. Transfer to bowls and serve hot.

Nutrition Facts Per Serving: Calories: 244; Fat: 2; Carbs: 38; Fiber: 6; Sugar: 4; Protein: 20

Broccoli Soup

(**Prep + Cook Time**: 30 minutes | **Servings**: 4)

Ingredients:
- 1 yellow onion; chopped
- 2 tbsp. olive oil
- 1 celery stick; chopped
- Zest from 1/2 lemon
- 1-quart veggie stock
- 17 oz. water
- 1 tsp. cumin; ground
- 1 broccoli head; florets separated
- Black pepper to the taste
- 3 garlic cloves; minced

- 2 bay leaves
- Juice of 1/2 lemon
- A pinch of sea salt

For the pesto:
- 1/2 cup almonds; chopped
- 1 garlic clove
- 2 tbsp. lemon juice
- 2 tbsp. olive oil
- 4 tbsp. green olives; pitted and chopped

Instructions:
1. Heat up a pot with 2 tbsp. olive oil over medium high heat, add onion, lemon zest and a pinch of salt, stir and cook for 3 minutes.
2. Add celery and 3 garlic cloves, stir and cook for 1 minute more.
3. Add stock, cumin, water and black pepper, stir; cover, bring to a boil and simmer for 10 minutes.
4. Add bay leaves and broccoli, stir; cover again and cook for 6 minutes more.
5. Take soup off the heat, discard bay leaves, transfer to your blender and pulse really well.
6. Add juice from 1/2 lemon, pulse again, return to the pot and heat up again over medium-low heat.
7. Meanwhile; in your food processor, blend well almond with 1 garlic clove, 2 tbsp. lemon juice, 2 tbsp. olive oil and green olives. Divide soup into bowls, top with the pesto you've just made and serve hot.

Nutrition Facts Per Serving: Calories: 139; Fat: 2; Fiber: 1; Carbs: 4; Protein: 1

Coconut And Zucchini Soup

(Prep + Cook Time: 25 minutes | **Servings:** 2)
Ingredients:
- 1 brown onion; chopped

- 1 tbsp. coconut oil
- 2 zucchinis; cubed
- A pinch of sea salt
- White pepper to the taste
- 2 tsp. turmeric powder
- 3 garlic cloves; chopped
- 1 tsp. curry powder
- 1 cup coconut milk
- 1 cup veggie stock
- 2 tbsp. lime juice
- Some chopped cilantro for serving

Instructions:

1. Heat up a pot with the oil over medium heat, add onion, stir and cook for 4 minutes.
2. Add garlic, salt, pepper and zucchinis, stir and cook for 1 minute.
3. Add turmeric and curry powder, stir well and cook for 1 minute more.
4. Add coconut milk and stock, stir; bring to a boil, cover pot and simmer soup for 10 minutes. Add lime juice and cilantro, stir; ladle into bowls and serve.

Nutritional value: Calories: 140; Fat: 1; Fiber: 1; Carbs: 2; Protein: 1

Special Chicken Soup

(**Prep + Cook Time**: 45 minutes | **Servings**: 6)

Ingredients:

- 2 celery stalks; chopped
- 1/2 cup coconut oil
- 2 carrots; chopped
- 1/2 cup arrowroot
- 6 cups chicken stock
- 1 tsp. dry parsley

- 1/2 cup water
- 1 bay leaf
- A pinch of sea salt
- Black pepper to the taste
- 1/2 tsp. dry thyme
- 1½ cups coconut milk
- 3 cups organic chicken meat; already cooked and cubed

Instructions:
1. Heat up a soup pot with the oil over medium-high heat, add carrots and celery, stir and cook for 10 minutes.
2. Add stock, stir and bring to a boil.
3. In a bowl; mix arrowroot with 1/2 cup water and whisk well.
4. Add this to soup and also add parsley, sea salt, pepper to the taste, bay leaf and thyme.
5. Stir and cook everything for 15 minutes. Add chicken meat and coconut milk, stir; cook 1 more minute, take off heat, pour into soup bowls and serve.

Nutrition Facts Per Serving: Calories: 412; Fat: 31; Carbs: 8; Fiber: 2; Protein: 27; Sugar: 4

Paleo Chicken Soup

(**Prep + Cook Time**: 25 minutes | **Servings**: 2)

Ingredients:
- 1 red bell pepper; chopped
- 1 tsp. coconut oil
- 1 yellow onion; chopped
- 1/4 cup pickled jalapeno peppers; chopped
- 2 garlic cloves; minced
- 1 tbsp. ghee
- 1 tsp. cumin; ground
- 1 tsp. coriander; ground
- 1 tsp. oregano; dried
- 1½ cups chicken breast; cooked and shredded

- 2½ cups chicken stock
- 2 cups kale; torn
- Zest from 1 lime; grated
- Juice from 1 lime
- A pinch of sea salt
- 15 oz. canned tomatoes; chopped
- 2 tbsp. spring onions; chopped
- 3 tbsp. pumpkin seeds; chopped
- 1 avocado; peeled, pitted and sliced
- 1 tsp. sweet paprika
- 3 tbsp. coriander; chopped

Instructions:
1. Heat up a pot with the oil over medium heat, add onion, stir and cook for 2 minutes.
2. Add red bell peppers, stir and cook for 1 minute. Add garlic, jalapenos, oregano, cumin, coriander and ghee, stir and cook for 1 minute more.
3. Add tomatoes, kale, chicken, lime zest, stock, lime juice and a pinch of salt, stir; bring to a boil, cook for 5 minutes and take off heat.
4. Heat up a pan over medium heat, add pumpkin seeds, toast them for 2 minutes and take off heat.
5. Ladle soup into bowls, top with pumpkin seeds, green onion, paprika, chopped coriander and avocado and serve.

Nutrition Facts Per Serving: Calories: 170; Fat: 2; Fiber: 3; Carbs: 4; Protein: 7

Paleo Nettles Soup

(**Prep + Cook Time**: 30 minutes | **Servings**: 3)
Ingredients:
- 1 tbsp. coconut oil
- 1 cup sweet potato; chopped
- 1 yellow onion; chopped
- 1/2 broccoli head; florets separated

- 1/2 cauliflower head; florets separated
- 1 bay leaf
- 3 garlic cloves; minced
- Zest from 1 lemon; grated
- 1 tsp. Dijon mustard
- 3½ cups veggie stock
- Black pepper to the taste
- A pinch of sea salt
- 4 cups nettles
- Juice of 1 lemon
- 5 thyme springs; leaves separated
- 4 bacon slices; cooked and crumbled
- 1/2 cup coconut cream

Instructions:
1. Heat up a pot with the coconut oil over medium heat, add sweet potato, onion, broccoli and cauliflower, stir and cook for 6 minutes.
2. Add bay leaf, garlic, veggie stock, lemon zest, salt, pepper and mustard, stir and bring to a boil.
3. Reduce heat, cover pot and cook for 10 minutes.
4. Meanwhile; put water in a pot and bring to a boil.
5. Cut nettles leaves with scissors, add leaves to water, leave there for 2 minutes, drain them and transfer them to the pot with the soup.
6. Cook for 3 minutes more, add lemon juice, blend using an immersion blender and then heat up the soup again.
7. Add thyme and coconut cream, stir; cook for 1 minute and ladle into soup bowls. Top with bacon and serve.

Nutrition Facts Per Serving: Calories: 170; Fat: 2; Fiber: 2; Carbs: 2; Protein: 8

Paleo Clam Soup

(**Prep + Cook Time**: 40 minutes | **Servings**: 6)
Ingredients:

- 1 small cauliflower head; florets separated
- 2 tbsp. coconut oil
- 2 cups chicken stock
- 2 carrots; chopped
- 1 onion; chopped
- 2 sweet potatoes; chopped
- 20 oz. canned clams
- 1 celery rib; chopped
- 1 cup coconut milk
- A pinch of sea salt
- Black pepper to the taste

Instructions:
1. Heat up a pot with half of the oil over medium high heat, add half of the onion, cauliflower and stock, stir; bring to a boil and cook for 10 minutes.
2. Use an immersion blender to make cream, transfer this to a bowl and leave aside for now.
3. Heat up the same pot with the rest of the oil over medium high heat, add the rest of the onion, celery, carrot, a pinch of sea salt and black pepper to the taste, stir and cook for 10 minutes.
4. Add potato, 2 cups of the cauliflower cream, stir; bring to a boil and simmer for 10 minutes.
5. Add coconut milk, clams and the rest of the cauliflower cream, stir and cook for 2 minutes more. Ladle into soup bowls and serve.

Nutrition Facts Per Serving: Calories: 250; Fat: 13; Fiber: 3; Carbs: 6; Protein: 12

Brussels Sprouts Soup

(**Prep + Cook Time**: 30 minutes | **Servings**: 4)
Ingredients:
- 2 tbsp. olive oil

- 1 yellow onion; chopped
- 2 lbs. Brussels sprouts; trimmed and halved
- 4 cups chicken stock
- 1/4 cup coconut cream
- A pinch of black pepper

Instructions:

1. Heat up a pot with the oil over medium high heat, add onion, stir and cook for 3 minutes.
2. Add Brussels sprouts, stir and cook for 2 minutes.
3. Add stock and black pepper, stir; bring to a simmer and cook for 20 minutes.
4. Use an immersion blender to make your cream, add coconut cream, stir well and ladle into bowls. Serve right away and serve.

Nutrition Facts Per Serving: Calories: 200; Fat: 11; Fiber: 3; Carbs: 6; Protein: 11

Squash Soup

(Prep + Cook Time: 60 minutes | **Servings**: 4)

Ingredients:

- 1 butternut squash; cut in halves lengthwise and deseeded
- 14 oz. coconut milk
- A pinch of sea salt
- Black pepper to the taste
- A handful parsley; chopped
- A pinch of nutmeg; ground

Instructions:

1. Place butternut squash halves on a lined baking sheet, place in the oven at 350 °F and bake for 45 minutes.
2. Leave squash to cool down, scoop flesh and transfer it to pot. Add half of the coconut milk and blend everything using an immersion blender.
3. Heat this soup up over medium-low heat, add the rest of the coconut milk, a pinch of sea salt, black pepper to the taste,

nutmeg and parsley, blend using your immersion blender for a few seconds, cook for about 4 minutes, divide into soup bowls and serve.

Nutrition Facts Per Serving: Calories: 144; Fat: 10; Fiber: 2; Carbs: 7; Protein: 2

Paleo Zucchini Soup

(**Prep + Cook Time**: 30 minutes | **Servings**: 4)

Ingredients:
- 1 onion; chopped
- 3 zucchinis; cut into medium chunks
- 2 tbsp. coconut milk
- 2 garlic cloves; minced
- 4 cups chicken stock
- 2 tbsp. coconut oil
- A pinch of sea salt
- Black pepper to the taste

Instructions:
1. Heat up a pot with the oil over medium heat, add zucchinis, garlic and onion, stir and cook for 5 minutes.
2. Add stock, salt, pepper, stir; bring to a boil, cover pot, simmer soup for 20 minutes and take off heat. Add coconut milk, blend using an immersion blender, ladle into bowls and serve.

Nutrition Facts Per Serving: Calories: 160; Fat: 2; Fiber: 2; Carbs: 4; Protein: 7

Tasty Mushroom Cream

(**Prep + Cook Time**: 30 minutes | **Servings**: 4)

Ingredients:
- 1 oz. dried porcini mushrooms
- 1 leek; chopped
- 2 tbsp. olive oil

- 1 celery stick; chopped
- 3 garlic cloves; chopped
- 14 brown mushrooms; chopped
- 1 tbsp. thyme; chopped
- 3 cups veggie stock
- 1 sweet potato; peeled and chopped
- 2 bay leaves
- 1/2 tsp. Dijon mustard
- 1 tsp. lemon zest; grated
- 1/2 tsp. black pepper
- 1 tbsp. lemon juice
- 3 tbsp. sunflower seed butter

Instructions:
1. Put dried mushrooms in a small bowl; cover with boiling water, leave aside for 10 minutes, strain, reserve water and chop them.
2. Heat up a pot with the oil over medium heat, add celery and leek, stir and cook for 5 minutes.
3. Add mushrooms, thyme, garlic and sweet potatoes, stir and cook for 1 minute.
4. Add dried mushrooms and half of their liquid, stock, bay leaves, mustard, black pepper and lemon zest, stir; cover pot and simmer soup over medium heat for 15 minutes.
5. Discard bay leaves, use an immersion blender to make your mushroom cream, add lemon juice and sunflower seed butter, stir well, ladle into bowls and serve.

Nutrition Facts Per Serving: Calories: 100; Fat: 2; Fiber: 1; Carbs: 4; Protein: 3

Veggie And Chorizo Stew

(**Prep + Cook Time**: 40 minutes | **Servings**: 3)
Ingredients:
- 1 yellow onion; chopped
- 1 tbsp. coconut oil

- 2 chorizo sausages; skinless and thinly sliced
- 1 red bell pepper; chopped
- 1 carrot; thinly sliced
- 1 celery stick; chopped
- 1 tomato; chopped
- 2 garlic cloves; finely minced
- 2 cups chicken broth
- 1 tbsp. lemon juice
- Black pepper to the taste
- 1 zucchini; chopped
- A handful parsley leaves; finely chopped

Instructions:

1. Heat up a pan with the oil over medium-high heat, add chorizo, onion, celery and carrot, stir and cook for 3 minutes.
2. Add red bell pepper, tomatoes and garlic, stir and cook 1 minute.
3. Add lemon juice, stock and pepper, stir; bring to a boil, cover pan, reduce heat to medium and cook for 10 minutes.
4. Add zucchini, stir; cover again and cook for 10 more minutes.
5. Uncover pan, cook the stew for 2 minutes more stirring often. Add parsley, stir; take off heat, transfer to dishes and serve.

Nutrition Facts Per Serving: Calories: 420; Fat: 12; Carbs: 45; Fiber: 11; Sugar: 5; Protein: 33.2

Paleo Cauliflower Cream

(**Prep + Cook Time**: 30 minutes | **Servings**: 2)

Ingredients:

- 1 yellow onion; chopped
- 2 tbsp. olive oil
- 1 cauliflower head; florets separated and chopped
- 3 cups veggie stock
- 3 garlic cloves; minced

- Black pepper to the taste
- A pinch of sea salt
- 3/4 cup bacon; chopped
- 1 tsp. coconut oil
- 1 egg
- 2 tbsp. cilantro; chopped

Instructions:

1. Heat up a pot with the olive oil over medium heat, add onion, stir and cook for 4 minutes.
2. Add stock, cauliflower and garlic, stir and bring to a boil.
3. Reduce heat to medium-low, season with a pinch of salt and black pepper to the taste, cover pot and simmer soup for 10 minutes.
4. Meanwhile; heat up a pan with the coconut oil over medium heat, add bacon, cook until it's crispy, transfer to paper towels, drain grease and leave aside for now.
5. Meanwhile; put water in a pot and bring to a boil.
6. Place a bowl on top of boiling water, crack the egg into the bowl; whisk it for 3 minutes and take off heat.
7. Take your cauliflower soup off the heat, blend it using an immersion blender, add whisked egg and blend some more. Ladle into bowls, sprinkle crumbled bacon and cilantro on top and serve.

Nutrition Facts Per Serving: Calories: 200; Fat: 3; Fiber: 2; Carbs: 4; Protein: 7

Eggplant Stew

(**Prep + Cook Time**: 40 minutes | **Servings**: 3)

Ingredients:

- 1 eggplant; chopped
- 1 yellow onion; chopped
- 2 tomatoes; chopped
- 1 tsp. cumin powder
- A pinch of sea salt

- Black pepper to the taste
- 1 cup tomato paste
- A pinch of cayenne pepper
- 1/2 cup water

Instructions:
1. Heat up a pan over medium-high heat, add water, tomato paste, a pinch of salt and pepper, cayenne and cumin and stir well.
2. Add the eggplant, tomato and onion, stir; bring to a boil, reduce heat to medium and cook for 30 minutes.
3. Take stew off heat, add a black pepper if needed, transfer to plates and serve.

Nutrition Facts Per Serving: Calories: 82; Fat: 0; Carbs: 16; Fiber: 1; Sugar: 0.5; Protein: 5

Easy Onion Soup

(**Prep + Cook Time**: 3 hours 10 minutes | **Servings**: 4)
Ingredients:
- 2 tbsp. avocado oil
- 5 yellow onions; cut into halves and then slice
- Black pepper to the taste
- 5 cups beef stock
- 3 thyme springs
- 1 tbsp. tomato paste

Instructions:
1. Heat up a pot with the oil over medium high heat, add onions and thyme, stir; reduce heat to low, cover and cook for 30 minutes.
2. Uncover the pot and cook onions for 1 hour and 30 minutes more stirring often.
3. Add tomato paste and stock, stir and simmer soup for 1 hour more. Ladle soup into bowls and serve.

Nutrition Facts Per Serving: Calories: 200; Fat: 4; Fiber: 4; Carbs: 6; Protein: 8

Cauliflower Soup

(**Prep + Cook Time**: 1 hour 10 minutes | **Servings**: 6)

Ingredients:
- 1 yellow onion; finely chopped
- 2 tbsp. extra virgin olive oil
- 2 lbs. cauliflower florets
- A pinch of sea salt
- Black pepper to the taste
- 20 saffron threads
- 2 garlic cloves; minced
- 5 cups veggie stock

Instructions:
1. Heat up a pot with the oil over medium heat, add onion and garlic, stir and cook for 10 minutes.
2. Add cauliflower, a pinch of sea salt and pepper to the taste, stir and cook for 12 more minutes.
3. Add stock, stir; bring to a boil, reduce heat to medium and simmer for 25 minutes.
4. Take soup off the heat, add saffron, cover pot and leave it aside for 20 minutes.
5. Transfer soup to your blender and pulse very well. Pour into soup bowls and serve right away.

Nutrition Facts Per Serving: Calories: 170; Fat: 11; Carbs: 5; Fiber: 2; Sugar: 0.1; Protein: 7

Awesome Seafood Soup

(**Prep + Cook Time**: 2 hours 40 minutes | **Servings**: 4)

Ingredients:
- 1 lb. cod fillets; cubed
- 10 garlic cloves; minced

- 3 tbsp. olive oil
- 1 tbsp. lemon juice
- 1/4 cup parsley; chopped
- 1 yellow onion; chopped
- 2 tomatoes; chopped
- 1 tbsp. tomato paste
- 2 bay leaves
- 2½ cups water
- A pinch of sea salt
- Black pepper to the taste
- 1 lb. shrimp; peeled and deveined
- 10 cherry tomatoes; halved
- 1 lb. mussels; scrubbed

Instructions:

1. In a bowl; mix 6 garlic cloves with 2 tbsp. oil, parsley and lemon juice and stir.
2. Add fish cubes, toss to coat, cover bowl and keep in the fridge for 2 hours.
3. Heat up a pot with the rest of the oil over medium high heat, add onion, stir and cook for 2 minutes.
4. Add the rest of the garlic, stir and cook for 1 minute.
5. Add tomatoes, tomato paste, bay leaves, water, salt, pepper and marinated fish, stir; bring to a simmer and cook for 10 minutes.
6. Add shrimp, cherry tomatoes and mussels, stir and cook for 6 minutes more. Discard unopened mussels, ladle soup into bowls and serve.

Nutrition Facts Per Serving: Calories: 160; Fat: 2; Fiber: 2; Carbs: 4; Protein: 7

Shrimp And Chicken Soup

(**Prep + Cook Time**: 40 minutes | **Servings**: 4)
Ingredients:

165

- 5 tbsp. curry paste
- 1 tbsp. coconut oil
- 1 big chicken breast; cut into thin strips
- 4 tbsp. coconut aminos
- 2 cups chicken stock
- Juice from 1 lime
- 1½ cups coconut milk
- 1 lb. shrimp; peeled and deveined
- 1/2 cup coconut cream
- A small broccoli head; florets separated
- 5 Chinese broccoli leaves; chopped
- 1 zucchini; chopped
- 1 carrot; chopped
- 1 cucumber; chopped
- Some chopped cilantro; chopped for serving

Instructions:
1. Heat up a pot with the oil over medium heat, add curry paste, stir and cook for 1 minute.
2. Add chicken, stir and cook for 1 minute more.
3. Add stock and lime juice, stir and cook for 2 minutes.
4. Add coconut cream, aminos and coconut milk, stir and cook for 10 minutes.
5. Add broccoli leaves, broccoli florets and carrots, stir and cook for 3 minutes.
6. Add shrimp and zucchini, stir and cook for 2 minutes. Ladle into bowls, top with cilantro and cucumber pieces and serve.

Nutritional value: Calories: 160; Fat: 3; Fiber: 2; Carbs: 6; Protein: 8

Paleo Sweet Potato Soup

(**Prep + Cook Time**: 35 minutes | **Servings**: 2)
Ingredients:
- 4 tbsp. olive oil

- 5 garlic cloves; minced
- 1 sweet potato; chopped
- 4 lemon peels
- 1/2 tsp. cumin seeds
- Black pepper to the taste
- 14 oz. veggie stock
- A pinch of sea salt
- 4 tbsp. pine nuts

Instructions:
1. Heat up a pot with the oil over medium heat, add garlic, stir and cook for 4 minutes.
2. Add lemon peel, sweet potato, stock, cumin, a pinch of salt and black pepper to the taste, stir; bring to a boil and cook for 15 minutes.
3. Heat up a pan over medium high heat, add pine nuts, stir and cook for 4 minutes.
4. Discard lemon peel from soup, blend it using an immersion blender and mix with half of the pine nuts. Blend again, ladle into bowls and sprinkle the rest of the pine nuts on top.

Nutrition Facts Per Serving: Calories: 150; Fat: 2; Fiber: 2; Carbs: 7; Protein: 3

Paleo Kale And Sausage Soup

(**Prep + Cook Time**: 45 minutes | **Servings**: 4)

Ingredients:
- 1 yellow onion; chopped
- 16 oz. sausage; chopped
- 3 sweet potatoes; chopped
- 4 cups chicken stock
- 1 lb. kale; chopped
- A pinch of sea salt and black pepper

Instructions:

1. Heat up a pot over medium heat, add sausage, stir; brown on both sides and transfer to a bowl.
2. Heat up the pot again over medium heat, add onion, stir and cook for 5 minutes.
3. Add stock and sweet potatoes, stir; bring to a simmer and cook for 20 minutes.
4. Use an immersion blender to blend your soup, add kale, a pinch of salt and black pepper and simmer everything for 2 minutes more. Ladle soup into bowls, top with sausage pieces and serve.

Nutrition Facts Per Serving: Calories: 200; Fat: 2; Fiber: 2; Carbs: 6; Protein: 8

Delicious Green Soup

(**Prep + Cook Time**: 35 minutes | **Servings**: 6)

Ingredients:
- 2 leeks; chopped
- 2 tbsp. ghee
- 4 celery sticks; chopped
- 4 garlic cloves; minced
- 2 broccoli heads; florets separated
- 1 small cauliflower head; florets separated
- 2 handfuls spinach; chopped
- 8 cups veggie stock
- 1 handful parsley; chopped
- 1 tbsp. coconut cream
- A pinch of nutmeg; ground
- Black pepper to the taste

Instructions:
1. Heat up a pot with the ghee over medium heat, add garlic and leeks, stir and cook for 3 minutes.
2. Add broccoli, celery and cauliflower, stir and cook for 5 minutes,
3. Add stock, bring to a boil, cover pot and cook for 15 minutes.

4. Add parsley and spinach, stir and blend using an immersion blender. Add black pepper and nutmeg, stir; ladle soup into bowls and serve with some coconut cream on top.

Nutrition Facts Per Serving: Calories: 103; Fat: 4; Fiber: 3; Carbs: 10; Protein: 4

Mexican Paleo Stew

(**Prep + Cook Time**: 60 minutes | **Servings**: 4)

Ingredients:
- 1 lb. beef meat; cubed
- 2 tbsp. avocado oil
- 1 tbsp. garlic; minced
- 1 brown onion; chopped
- 1 bay leaf
- 1 Serrano pepper; chopped
- 1 tsp. chili powder
- 1 tsp. cumin; ground
- 1 tsp. paprika
- Black pepper to the taste
- 1/2 tsp. oregano; dried
- 1/2 tsp. chipotle powder
- 1 cup chicken stock
- 1 tbsp. tapioca flour
- 1/2 cup tomato sauce

Instructions:
1. Set you pressure cooker on Sauté mode, add oil, heat it up, add beef, stir and brown for a few minutes on each side.
2. Add garlic, Serrano pepper, onion, bay leaf, black pepper, paprika, chili powder, cumin, oregano and chipotle powder, stir and cook for 4 minutes more.
3. Add stock, tapioca flour and tomato sauce, stir; cover pot and cook on High for 35 minutes. Release the pressure, uncover, stir you stew one more time and serve right away.

Nutrition Facts Per Serving: Calories: 300; Fat: 12; Fiber: 3; Carbs: 6; Protein: 17

Tasty Turkey Soup

(**Prep + Cook Time**: 40 minutes | **Servings**: 4)

Ingredients:

- 3½ cups chicken stock
- 3 tbsp. coconut oil
- 1 cup coconut cream
- 3 celery stalks; chopped
- 2 carrots; chopped
- 1 sweet potato; peeled and cubed
- 2 cups turkey meat; cooked and shredded
- 1 yellow onion; chopped
- 1 tbsp. sage; chopped
- 1 tsp. thyme; dried
- A handful parsley; chopped
- Black pepper to the taste
- A pinch of sea salt

Instructions:

1. Heat up a pot with the oil over medium heat, add celery, onions, sweet potato and carrots, stir and cook for 5 minutes.
2. Add stock, a pinch of salt, black pepper to the taste, stir; bring to a simmer and cook for 20 minutes.
3. Add turkey, coconut cream, sage, parsley and thyme, stir; cook for 2 minutes more, ladle into bowls and serve.

Nutrition Facts Per Serving: Calories: 180; Fat: 3; Fiber: 2; Carbs: 3; Protein: 5

Celery Soup

(**Prep + Cook Time**: 30 minutes | **Servings**: 2)

Ingredients:

- 2 tbsp. cashews; chopped

- 17 oz. veggie stock
- A pinch of sea salt
- Black pepper to the taste
- 1½ tbsp. olive oil
- 1 yellow onion; chopped
- 13 oz. celery; chopped

Instructions:

1. Heat up a pot with the oil over medium high heat, add onion and celery, stir and cook for 5 minutes.
2. Add stock, a pinch of salt and black pepper to the taste, stir; bring to a simmer and cook for 10 minutes.
3. Add cashews, stir and cook for 5 minutes more. Transfer this to your blender, pulse really well until you obtain cream, divide into bowls and serve.

Nutrition Facts Per Serving: Calories: 150; Fat: 2; Fiber: 2; Carbs: 4; Protein: 7

Yummy Veggie Soup

(**Prep + Cook Time**: 25 minutes | **Servings**: 4)

Ingredients:

- 1 yellow onion; chopped
- 2 carrots; chopped
- 6 mushrooms; chopped
- 1 red chili pepper; chopped
- 2 celery sticks; chopped
- 1 tbsp. coconut oil
- A pinch of sea salt
- Black pepper to the taste
- A handful dried porcini mushrooms
- 4 garlic cloves; minced
- 4 oz. kale; chopped
- 1 cup canned tomatoes; chopped
- 1 zucchini; chopped

- 1-quart veggie stock
- 1 bay leaf
- Some lemon zest; grated for serving
- A handful parsley; chopped for serving

Instructions:
1. Set your instant pot on Sauté mode, add oil and heat it up.
2. Add celery, carrots, onion, a pinch of salt and black pepper, stir and cook for 2 minutes.
3. Add chili pepper, garlic, dried mushrooms and mushrooms, stir and cook for 2 minutes.
4. Add tomatoes, stock, bay leaf, kale and zucchinis, stir; cover pot and cook on High for 10 minutes. Release pressure, stir soup again, ladle into bowls, top with lemon zest and parsley and serve.

Nutrition Facts Per Serving: Calories: 150; Fat: 2; Fiber: 2; Carbs: 4; Protein: 6

Delicious Pork Stew

(**Prep + Cook Time**: 8 hours 10 minutes | **Servings**: 8)

Ingredients:
- 2 lbs. pork loin; cubed and marinated in some beer in the fridge for 1 day
- 1 tbsp. coconut oil
- 3 garlic cloves; minced
- 1 cup arrowroot flour
- 6 carrots; chopped
- Black pepper to the taste
- A pinch of sea salt
- 2 yellow onions; chopped
- 1 small cabbage head; finely chopped
- 5 small sweet potatoes; chopped
- 30 oz. canned tomatoes; chopped
- 3 cups beef stock

Instructions:

1. In a bowl mix arrowroot flour with marinated pork cubes and rub them well.
2. Heat up a pan with the oil over medium high heat, add pork cubes, brown them on all sides and transfer to your slow cooker.
3. Add garlic, carrots, a pinch of salt, black pepper, onion, cabbage, sweet potatoes, tomatoes and stock, stir; cover pot and cook your stew on Low for 8 hours. Uncover pot, stir stew again, divide into bowls and serve.

Nutrition Facts Per Serving: Calories: 260; Fat: 6; Fiber: 4; Carbs: 7; Protein: 14

Delightful Beef Stew

(**Prep + Cook Time**: 8 hours 10 minutes | **Servings**: 4)

Ingredients:

- 2½ lbs. beef chuck; cubed
- 3 cups collard greens
- 3 cups water
- 5 green plantains; peeled and cubed
- 3 tbsp. allspice
- 1/4 cup garlic powder
- 1/3 cup sweet paprika
- 1 tsp. cayenne pepper
- 1 tsp. chili powder

Instructions:

1. In your slow cooker, mix beef with greens, plantains, water, allspice, garlic powder, paprika, cayenne and chili powder, stir well, cover and cook on Low for 8 hours.
2. Keep stirring from time to time. Divide into bowls and serve.

Nutrition Facts Per Serving: Calories: 250; Fat: 4; Fiber: 3; Carbs: 5; Protein: 9

Simple Roasted Veggie Stew

(Prep + Cook Time: 1 hour 10 minutes | **Servings**: 6)

Ingredients:

- 1 garlic head; cloves peeled
- 4 lbs. mixed parsnips; carrots, turnips and celery root, peeled and roughly chopped
- 1/2 cup yellow onion; chopped
- 6 tbsp. olive oil
- 1 tbsp. tomato paste
- 28 oz. canned tomatoes; chopped
- A pinch of sea salt
- Black pepper to the taste
- 2 cups kale; chopped
- 1 tsp. oregano; dried

Instructions:

1. In a big baking dish, mix root veggies with garlic cloves, half of the oil, a pinch of salt and pepper, toss to coat, place in the oven at 450 °F and roast for 45 minutes.
2. Heat up a pan with the rest of the oil over medium high heat, add onion, stir and cook for 3 minutes.
3. Add tomato paste, stir and cook for 1 minute.
4. Add canned tomatoes, oregano and some black pepper, stir; bring to a simmer and cook for a few minute more.
5. Take veggies out of the oven and add them to the pot with the tomatoes.
6. Also add kale, stir and cook everything for 5 minutes. Divide into bowls and serve.

Nutrition Facts Per Serving: Calories: 200; Fat: 3; Fiber: 3; Carbs: 5; Protein: 5

Slow Cooked Paleo Stew

(Prep + Cook Time: 7 hours 10 minutes | **Servings**: 4)

Ingredients:

- 2 tbsp. olive oil
- 8 carrots; chopped
- 2 parsnips; chopped
- 1½ lbs. beef meat; cubed
- 2 bay leaves
- 1/2 tsp. peppercorns
- 1 yellow onion; chopped
- 1/4 cup tapioca flour
- 1 tbsp. thyme; chopped
- 2 tbsp. water
- 4 cups beef stock
- A pinch of sea salt
- Black pepper to the taste

Instructions:

1. Heat up a pan with the oil over medium high heat, add beef, stir; brown for 4 minutes on all sides and transfer to your slow cooker.
2. Add peppercorns, parsnips, carrots, onion, bay leaves, thyme, stock, a pinch of salt and black pepper, stir; cover and cook on High for 6 hours and 30 minutes.
3. Uncover slow cooker, add tapioca mixed with the water, stir; cover again and cook on High for 30 minutes more. Uncover pot again, discard bay leaves, divide stew into bowls and serve.

Nutrition Facts Per Serving: Calories: 200; Fat: 5; Fiber: 3; Carbs: 4; Protein: 8

Tasty Chicken Stew

(**Prep + Cook Time**: 8 hours 10 minutes | **Servings**: 6)

Ingredients:

- 2 carrots; chopped
- 5 garlic cloves; minced
- 2 celery sticks; chopped

- 2 onions; chopped
- 2 sweet potatoes; cubed
- 30 oz. canned pumpkin puree
- 2 quarts chicken stock
- 2 cups chicken meat; skinless, boneless and shredded
- A pinch of sea salt
- Black pepper to the taste
- 1/4 tsp. cayenne pepper
- 1/4 cup arrowroot powder
- 1/2 lb. baby spinach

Instructions:

1. In your slow cooker, mix carrots with garlic, celery, onion, sweet potatoes, pumpkin puree, chicken, stock, salt, pepper, cayenne and arrowroot powder, stir; cover and cook on Low for 7 hours and 40 minutes.
2. Uncover slow cooker, add spinach, cover again and cook on Low for 20 minutes more. Divide into bowls and serve.

Nutrition Facts Per Serving: Calories: 280; Fat: 3; Fiber: 3; Carbs: 6; Protein: 7

Yummy Cucumber Soup

(**Prep + Cook Time**: 2 hours 10 minutes | **Servings**: 2)

Ingredients:

- 2 cucumbers; chopped
- 1 cup coconut cream
- 1 garlic clove; minced
- 1 tbsp. olive oil
- 3 tbsp. lemon juice
- A pinch of sea salt
- Black pepper to the taste

Instructions:

1. In your food processor, blend cucumber with a pinch of sea salt and black pepper, coconut cream, garlic, oil and lemon

juice and pulse really well. Divide into soup bowls and serve cold.

Nutrition Facts Per Serving: Calories: 120; Fat: 1; Fiber: 1; Carbs: 3; Protein: 1

French Style Chicken Stew

(**Prep + Cook Time**: 2 hours 10 minutes | **Servings**: 4)

Ingredients:
- 10 garlic cloves
- 2 lbs. chicken pieces
- 30 oz. canned tomatoes; chopped
- 30 black olives; pitted and chopped
- 2 cups chicken stock
- 2 tbsp. parsley; chopped
- 2 tbsp. thyme; chopped
- 2 tbsp. basil; chopped
- 2 tbsp. coconut oil
- A pinch of sea salt
- Black pepper to the taste
- 2 tbsp. rosemary; chopped

Instructions:
1. Heat up a pot with the oil over medium high heat, add chicken pieces, season with a pinch of salt and black pepper to the taste, stir and brown them for 2 minutes on each side.
2. Add garlic, stock, thyme, tomatoes, olives, rosemary, basil and parsley, stir; cover, place in the oven at 325 °F and bake for 2 hours. Divide into bowls and serve.

Nutrition Facts Per Serving: Calories: 240; Fat: 10; Fiber: 4; Carbs: 6; Protein: 24

Special Paleo Stew

(**Prep + Cook Time**: 8 hours 10 minutes | **Servings**: 6)

Ingredients:
- 1 cup carrots; chopped
- 1 cup celery; chopped

- 2 cups onions; chopped
- 3 lbs. osso buco; bones in
- 4 garlic cloves; minced
- 6 tsp. baharat
- A pinch of black pepper
- 2 cups beef stock
- A handful parsley; chopped
- 1 kale; chopped

Instructions:

1. In your slow cooker, mix osso buco with carrots, celery, onions, garlic, baharat, black pepper and stock, stir; cover and cook on Low for 7 hours and 30 minutes.
2. Uncover your slow cooker, add kale and parsley, cover again and cook for 30 minutes more. Divide stew into bowls and serve.

Nutrition Facts Per Serving: 340; Fat: 2; Fiber: 3; Carbs: 4; Protein: 10

Lamb And Coconut Stew

(**Prep + Cook Time**: 2 hours 5 minutes | **Servings**: 4)

Ingredients:

- 1½ lbs. lamb meat; diced
- 1 tbsp. coconut oil
- 1/2 red chili; seedless and chopped
- 1 brown onion; chopped
- 3 garlic cloves; minced
- 2 celery sticks; chopped
- 2½ tsp. garam masala powder
- 1 tsp. fennel seeds
- A pinch of sea salt
- Black pepper to the taste
- 1¼ tsp. turmeric
- 1½ tsp. ghee

- 14 oz. canned coconut milk
- 1 cup water
- 1 tbsp. lemon juice
- 2 carrots; chopped
- A handful parsley leaves; finely chopped

Instructions:
1. Heat up a pan with the oil over medium-high heat, add lamb, stir and brown for 4 minutes.
2. Add celery, chili and onion, stir and cook 1 minute.
3. Reduce heat to medium, add garam masala, garlic, ghee, fennel and turmeric, stir and cook 1 minute.
4. Add a pinch of sea salt, pepper to the taste, tomato paste, coconut milk and water, stir; bring to a boil, reduce heat to low, cover and cook for 1 hour.
5. Add carrots and cook for 40 minutes more, stirring from time to time. Add lemon juice and parsley, stir; take off heat, transfer to bowls and serve.

Nutrition Facts Per Serving: Calories: 450; Fat: 31; Carbs: 40; Fiber: 1; Sugar: 2; Protein: 50

Yummy Slow Cooker Stew

(**Prep + Cook Time**: 32 hours | **Servings**: 6)

Ingredients:
- 2 lbs. beef stew meat; cubed
- 3 cups dark beer
- 7 garlic cloves; finely minced
- A pinch of sea salt
- Black pepper to the taste
- 4 carrots; chopped
- 1 cup coconut flour
- 2 yellow onions; finely chopped
- 1/2 head cabbage; finely chopped

- 30 oz. canned tomatoes; diced
- 2 cups reserved beef marinade
- 3 cups beef stock

Instructions:

1. In a bowl; mix beef with beer and 3 garlic cloves, toss to coat and keep in the fridge for 1 day.
2. In a bowl; mix coconut flour with a pinch of sea salt and pepper to the taste and stir.
3. Drain meat and reserve the 2 cups of the marinade.
4. Add meat to tapioca bowls and toss to coat.
5. Heat up a pan over medium-high heat, add meat, stir and brown it for 2-3 minutes.
6. Transfer meat to your slow cooker.
7. Add reserved marinade, carrots, cabbage, onions, tomatoes, 4 garlic cloves, beef stock, salt and pepper to the taste, cover pot and cook stew on Low for 8 hours. Uncover pot, transfer stew to bowls and serve.

Nutrition Facts Per Serving: Calories: 247; Fat: 4.5; Carbs: 25; Fiber: 4.2; Sugar: 4; Protein: 24.2

Paleo Asparagus Soup

(**Prep + Cook Time**: 35 minutes | **Servings**: 3)

Ingredients:

- 1 celery stick; chopped
- 1 zucchini; chopped
- 1 yellow onion; chopped
- 2 lbs. asparagus; trimmed and roughly chopped
- 2 garlic cloves; minced
- Grated lemon peel from 1/2 lemon
- Black pepper to the taste
- 2 cups water
- 1 tbsp. olive oil

Instructions:

1. Place asparagus, zucchini, celery, onion, lemon peel and garlic on a lined baking sheet, drizzle the oil, season with

black pepper, place in the oven at 400 °F and bake for 25 minutes.
2. Transfer these to a food processor, add the water and pulse really well.
3. Transfer soup to a pot and heat up over medium high heat. Ladle into bowls and serve right away.

Nutrition Facts Per Serving: Calories: 160; Fat: 3; Fiber: 2; Carbs: 6; Protein: 6

Tasty Beef Stew

(**Prep + Cook Time**: 2 hours 40 minutes | **Servings**: 4)

Ingredients:
- 2 lbs. beef meat; cubed
- 3 yellow onions; chopped
- Black pepper to the taste
- 2 tbsp. Moroccan spices
- 1/3 cup ghee
- 2 cups beef stock
- 3 garlic cloves; minced
- 1 lemon; sliced
- Juice of 1 lemon
- Zest from 1 lemon; grated
- 1 butternut squash; peeled, seeded and cubed
- 1 bunch cilantro; chopped

Instructions:
1. Heat up a Dutch ovenn with the ghee over medium heat, add beef, onions, spices, black pepper, garlic, lemon slices, lemon juice and zest and stock, stir; place in the oven at 300 °F and cook for 2 hours.
2. Add cilantro and squash, stir and cook in the oven for 30 minutes more. Divide into bowls and serve.

Nutrition Facts Per Serving: Calories: 300; Fat: 12; Fiber: 3; Carbs: 6; Protein: 17

Paleo Vietnamese Stew

(Prep + Cook Time: 3 hours 30 minutes | **Servings**: 6)

Ingredients:
- 1 lemongrass stalk; chopped
- 2½ lbs. organic beef brisket; cut into medium chunks
- 1½ tsp. curry powder
- 2½ tbsp. ginger; grated
- 2 tbsp. unsweetened applesauce
- 3 tbsp. ghee
- 1 bay leaf
- 1 yellow onion; chopped
- 2-star anise
- 2 cups canned tomatoes; chopped
- 3 cups water
- 1 lb. carrots; chopped
- 1/4 cup cilantro; chopped
- A pinch of sea salt
- Black pepper to the taste

Instructions:
1. In a bowl; mix applesauce with lemongrass, curry powder, bay leaf, ginger and beef, toss to coat well and leave aside for 30 minutes.
2. Heat up a pot with the ghee over medium high heat, add beef, stir; brown on all sides and transfer to a plate.
3. Add marinade to browned beef and toss again.
4. Return pot to medium heat, add onion, stir and cook for a few minutes.
5. Add a pinch of salt, black pepper and tomatoes, stir and cook for 15 minutes.
6. Add beef and its marinade and star anise, stir and cook for 5 minutes.
7. Add carrots and water, stir; bring to a boil, cover, place in the oven at 300 degrees and bake for 2 hours and 30 minutes.

8. Discard bay leaf and star anise, stir the stew, divide into bowls, sprinkle cilantro on top and serve.

Nutrition Facts Per Serving: Calories: 300; Fat: 4; Fiber: 3; Carbs: 6; Protein: 12

African Style Stew

(**Prep + Cook Time**: 55 minutes | **Servings**: 4)

Ingredients:
- 4 chicken thighs
- 1 small brown onion; chopped
- 1/2 tbsp. coconut oil
- A pinch of sea salt
- Black pepper to the taste
- 1 tbsp. ginger; grated
- 1 tbsp. garlic; minced
- 1/2 tsp. paprika
- 1/2 tbsp. coriander
- 1/2 tsp. chili powder
- 2 cloves
- 2 bay leaves
- 1½ cups canned tomatoes; chopped
- 2½ tbsp. cashew butter
- 1/4 cup water
- 1 tbsp. parsley; chopped
- 1/4 tsp. vanilla extract

Instructions:
1. Heat up a pan with the oil over medium high heat, add chicken pieces, season with a pinch of salt and black pepper to the taste, stir; brown for 4 minutes on each side and transfer them to a bowl.
2. Heat up the same pan over medium heat, add ginger and onion, stir and cook for 6 minutes.

3. Add garlic, paprika, coriander, bay leaves, cloves and chili powder, stir and cook for 1 minute.
4. Add water, tomatoes and chicken pieces, stir; cover, bring to a boil and simmer for 25 minutes.
5. Take chicken out of the pot, add cashew butter and vanilla, stir and cook for 2 minutes more. Divide chicken into bowls, add stew on top, sprinkle parsley and serve hot.

Nutrition Facts Per Serving: Calories: 200; Fat: 4; Fiber: 2; Carbs: 5; Protein: 8

Yummy Chorizo Stew

(**Prep + Cook Time**: 40 minutes | **Servings**: 3)
Ingredients:
- 1 carrot; chopped
- 1 yellow onion; chopped
- 1 tbsp. coconut oil
- 2 chorizo sausages; chopped
- 1 red bell pepper; chopped
- 1 celery stick; chopped
- 2 sweet potatoes; chopped
- 2 garlic cloves; minced
- 1 tomato; chopped
- 2 cups chicken stock
- A handful parsley; chopped
- 1 zucchini; chopped
- 1 tbsp. lemon juice
- A pinch of sea salt
- Black pepper to the taste

Instructions:
1. Heat up a pan with the oil over medium high heat, add carrot, onion, chorizo and celery, stir and cook for 3 minutes.
2. Add sweet potatoes, garlic, tomato and red bell pepper, stir and cook for 1 minute more.

3. Add lemon juice, a pinch of salt, black pepper and stock, stir; cover, bring to a simmer and cook for 10 minutes.
4. Add zucchini, stir and cook for 12 minutes more. Add parsley, stir well, divide into bowls and serve.

Nutrition Facts Per Serving: Calories: 270; Fat: 8; Fiber: 3; Carbs: 5; Protein: 8

Paleo Oxtail Stew

(**Prep + Cook Time**: 6 hours 10 minutes | **Servings**: 8)

Ingredients:
- 5 lbs. oxtail; cut into medium chunks
- 2 celery stick; chopped
- 2 leeks; chopped
- A pinch of sea salt
- Black pepper to the taste
- 2 tbsp. avocado oil
- 3 thyme springs
- 4 carrots; chopped
- 3 rosemary springs
- 2 tbsp. coconut flour
- 4 cloves
- 4 bay leaves
- 28 oz. canned tomatoes; chopped
- 1-quart beef stock

Instructions:
1. Place oxtail in a roasting pan, season with a pinch of salt and black pepper, drizzle half of the avocado oil, rub well, place in the oven at 425 °F and roast for 20 minutes.
2. Heat up a pan with the rest of the oil over medium heat, add leeks, carrots, celery, thyme, rosemary and bay leaf, stir and cook for 20 minutes.
3. Add coconut flour, cloves, tomatoes and stock and stir.

4. Add oxtail, stir; cover pan and cook on low heat for 5 hours. Take oxtail out of the pot, discard bones, return them to the pot, stir; divide into bowls and serve.

Nutrition Facts Per Serving: Calories: 435; Fat: 23; Fiber: 3; Carbs: 7; Protein: 30

Hearty Meat Paleo Stew

(**Prep + Cook Time**: 4 hours 10 minutes | **Servings**: 8)

Ingredients:
- 2 leeks; chopped
- 2 yellow onions; chopped
- 2 bay leaves
- 1 carrot; chopped
- 3 garlic cloves; minced
- 1½ tsp. thyme; chopped
- 3 cups veggie stock
- 1 tbsp. lemon juice
- 3 tbsp. parsley; chopped
- Black pepper to the taste
- A pinch of sea salt
- 1 lb. beef chuck; cubed
- 1 lb. pork butt; cubed
- 1 lb. lamb shoulder; cubed
- 3 sweet potatoes; cubed
- 1 tbsp. coconut oil
- 3 bacon slices

Instructions:
1. In a Dutch oven, mix leeks with onions, bay leaves, carrot, garlic, thyme, parsley, lemon juice, beef, pork, lamb, a pinch of salt and black pepper to the taste and toss to coat
2. Add oil, potatoes and top with bacon, place in the oven at 350 °F and bake for 4 hours. Divide into bowls and serve.

Nutrition Facts Per Serving: Calories: 340; Fat: 9; Fiber: 5; Carbs: 7; Protein: 15

Paleo Beef And Sweet Potatoes Stew

(**Prep + Cook Time**: 45 minutes | **Servings**: 4)

Ingredients:

- 1 red onion; chopped
- 1 tbsp. balsamic vinegar
- 2 tbsp. coconut oil
- A pinch of sea salt
- 1 lb. beef; ground
- 1/4 cup pine nuts
- 3 garlic cloves; minced
- 2/3 tsp. ginger; grated
- 1 tsp. coriander seeds
- 1 tsp. cumin; ground
- 1 tsp. paprika
- 3 cups sweet potatoes; peeled and cubed
- 1½ cups veggie stock
- 1 carrot; chopped
- 2/3 cup canned tomatoes; chopped
- 1/4 cup parsley; chopped
- Zest from 1 lemon; grated

Instructions:

1. Heat up a pot with the oil over medium heat, add onion and a pinch of salt, stir and cook for 10 minutes.
2. Add vinegar, stir and cook for 1 minute more.
3. Heat up another pan over medium heat, add pine nuts, stir; toast for 2 minutes and transfer to a bowl.
4. Add ginger and meat to onions, stir and cook for 2 minutes.
5. Add garlic, coriander, cumin and paprika, stir and cook for 2 minutes.

6. Add pine nuts, stock, carrot, tomatoes and lemon zest, stir; cover and cook for 20 minutes. Add parsley, stir; cook for 2 minutes more, divide into bowls and serve.

Nutrition Facts Per Serving: Calories: 200; Fat: 5; Fiber: 3; Carbs: 6; Protein: 10

www.ingramcontent.com/pod-product-compliance
Lightning Source LLC
Chambersburg PA
CBHW060323030426
42336CB00011B/1174